gorgeous to go

The Beaut.ie guide to smart shopping

About the author

Aisling McDermott set up Beaut.ie,
The Irish Beauty Blog, with her sister
Kirstie in 2006. Updated five times daily, it is the number one
Irish resource for information about make-up, skincare, hair
care, nails and just about anything connected with beauty
you can think of. Aisling lives with her husband and her
three British Shorthair cats.

gorgeous to go

The Beaut.ie guide to smart shopping

AISLING McDERMOTT

Gill & Macmillan

Gill & Macmillan

Hume Ave, Park West, Dublin 12

With associated companies throughout the world

www.gillmacmillan.ie

978 07171 4865 3

Index compiled by Kate Murphy

Print origination and design by Design Image

Printed in Italy by L.E.G.O. SpA

This book is typeset in Agenda

The paper used in this book comes from the wood pulp of managed forests.

For every tree felled, at least one tree is planted, thereby renewing natural

resources.

Photo credits:

For permission to reproduce photographs, the author and publisher gratefully

acknowledge the following: © Shutterstock: pp. 1, 8, 19, 64, 69, 74, 78, 80, 89, 90,

96, 101, 107, 108, 118, 124, 141, 152, 174, 196 and 204.

Contents

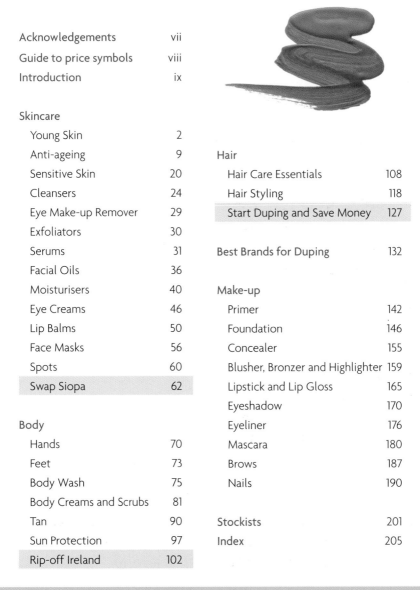

Acknowledgements

I would like to thank so many people who have laughed with me, put up with my lightning hoor ways, my inability to be on time, ever, and my general dizziness (included in this is never remembering to charge my mobile or reply to e-mails). It is only because of my strong supporting cast that I am actually able to do things like write this book. So starring in my acknowledgements are:

My sister Kirstie. I love her to bits and want to take this opportunity to declare my thanks for everything she's done to make this all possible. She's the hardest-working person I've ever met and the one who knows the most about lipstick in the world. Yes, the whole world. She is possibly the funniest person you could ever meet too. I only have to hear that dirty laugh across a crowded room and I know the party's right here.

Derrick, my handsome husband who knows more about make-up than any man ever wanted to but bears the strain of the knowledge admirably – thank you for it all (not just the book); Michelle, my best friend since we were chislers, for her love and support; Faith, agent to the stars and also to me; Lauren, also fabulous agent; Roísín, the famous one who has all the ideas; Donal Costigan; Ellen Breen, Mum, endless support and fun; Dad, endless ferrying me around and so kind; Shauna, endless positivity and help with proofing; and lovely Sarah, Fergal, Peter, Nikki, Teresa and everyone in Gill & Macmillan for their support and encouragement.

The Beaut.ies – you're deadly, all of you. We've had so much fun over the years and you've contributed your wisdom to this book in so many ways. Keep on commenting!

And all the friends I've made along the way; all the *craic* I've had, the drinks I've drank and the laughs we've had. This book is (sniffs back tears, getting all sentimental now and about to break into a *sean nós*) for you all.

Aisling x

Guide to the price symbols used in this book

To give you an idea of the price of products before you head to the shops, we've flagged each one with these symbols.

€	less than €10
€€	€10–€20
€€€	€21–€30
€€€€	€31–€40
€€€€€	€41–€50
€€€€€+	over €50

If you use this book properly, you'll soon find that you can pick up products for less than these guideline prices – checking for two for one offers, sales, buy one get one free (BOGOF) and gift with purchase (GWP) will soon become second nature to you.

All prices are based on RRPs and are correct at the time of going to press.

Premium brand: Think of a high-end cosmetic brand that you can buy in a department store. Estée Lauder, Chanel and MAC are examples.

Own brand: The big supermarkets and chemists all produce their own skincare or cosmetic lines, such as Tesco, Boots and Aldi.

Introduction

This book evolved with the telling. I had originally planned to write a straightforward shopping companion to *The Beaut.ie Guide to Gorgeous*, a handbag guide to what's great and worth buying.

Well, this book is still a handy guide to bring to the shops, of course – it's stuffed full of recommendations and tips – but it's become much more than that. When the economy seriously tanked and the IMF moved in, we as a nation became armchair economists like never before. People became obsessed with saving money and seeking out value, particularly in areas that might be considered non-essential.

But it's a mistake to think that beauty spending is a non-essential. Women regard spending on beauty as so essential that they will trade down in other areas in order to keep their make-up habit going – a trend that's been documented through many recessions. When Irish women began to seek better value in cosmetics, we introduced the Beaut.ienomics section on the website in response. We review products that are great value, highlight special offers and write about cases of downright bad value too.

The beauty industry in Ireland is huge and operates just like any other industry where Big Money is concerned. All sorts of tricks are employed to get you to part with as much cash as possible. This book tells you about them so you know what to look for – and also tells you what's worth buying.

Here are a few ways you can start to use the information in this book straightaway to save money and seek better value.

- Stop being so brand loyal – it's possible to swap out products for much less pricey alternatives. Cosmetics at the lower end of the scale have improved in leaps and bounds and it's possible to buy really good skincare and make-up for a fraction of the price of high-end brands. This book will tell you what's worth your money.

- Start duping. This is the best way to start shaking up your brand loyalty and is something you might not have even thought of doing before. It's also a great way to see what other people are rating. This trend originated on American beauty blogs and we've got tons of recommendations for you on Beaut.ie and in this book to get you started (see pp. 127–35 for more on duping).
- Stockpile when you see buy one get one free (BOGOF) offers, discounts, loyalty card bonus offers or three for two offers. Shampoo, shower gel and deodorant are all things that we need to buy constantly and you'll often see them in this kind of offer.
- Don't believe the hype! Words like 'luminosity' don't actually mean anything and anyone can give their product a name that sounds a bit like Botox, but that doesn't mean it will freeze your wrinkles. (It won't, by the way.) Instead, get recommendations to make sure the product is actually any good before you buy.
- Always try to get the best deal. That might mean shopping online, using a beauty loyalty card like those offered by Debenhams or Boots or snapping up gift sets post-Christmas.
- Shop with cash. You'll be less tempted to spend money you don't have and your credit card balance will thank you.
- Help us to put pressure on the cosmetics industry to get better value. Join Beaut.ie and sign our online petition to lower cosmetic prices in Ireland. We pay more for cosmetics than almost every other country in the world and it is an absolute disgrace that this situation exists. Anyone who shops online in the UK or the US knows that Ireland is a black spot for cosmetic pricing. You'll find our campaign at www.beaut.ie.

I hope you enjoy this book as much as I enjoyed writing it and use it to save tons of money and fall in love with some great products!

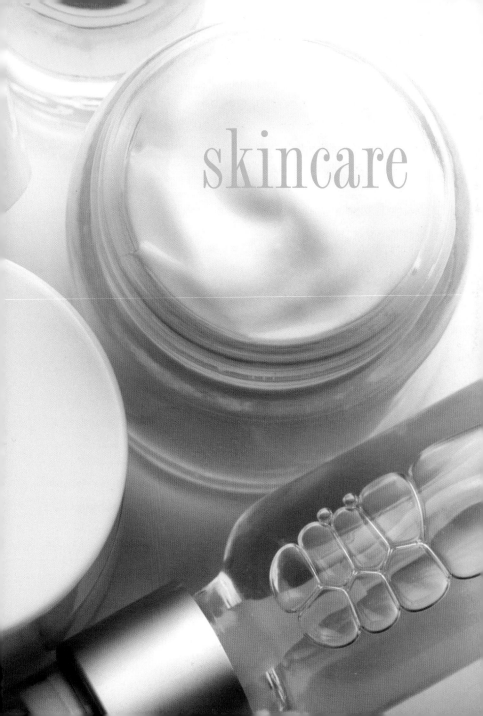

Young Skin

Young skin (and by this we mean anything from pre-teen to mid-twenties) has its own specific concerns. Skin can seem to go bonkers during the teenage years and hormonal changes can cause untold misery with spots, blackheads and oily patches all seeming to conspire to ruin your life, particularly when they conspire on the day of the debs or immediately before the disco where HE might finally notice you.

Unfortunately, he won't notice you if you spend the night sobbing in the jacks about the huge crop of blackheads that's just sprung up on your nose, that's for sure.

The good news is that cosmetic companies have copped on to this in a big way and are now producing good-quality products for teenage and early twenty-something skin. Of course they're not doing this out of the goodness of their hearts. You are a group with increasing purchasing power and we are image conscious in Ireland from a very early age.

But it doesn't really matter why they're doing it, does it? Having great skin is something that everyone wants — and here are some products that will help you to get it.

Beaut.ienomics: Double Up

We're seeing a big trend for multifunctional products in this category, which is excellent because as well as a cleanser you'll also get a product that exfoliates at the same time, and that will only save you time and money. Look for products like L'Oréal Paris Scrublet.

Beaut.ienomics:
Tweens and Pester Power

We're all familiar with the power of pester — it's just a nice phrase to describe the power of nagging, screaming and tantrum throwing.

The tear-soaked pester power story begins at toddler age with the sweets placed enticingly at the till at the supermarket and includes the whole of Smyths toy store and half the Argos catalogue. Aided and abetted by advertising, it nimbly progresses up to the tween age group (nine to 12 years) without pausing for breath. By now, anything with Hannah Montana and Justin Bieber plastered on them are objects of desire that must be purchased right now. Immediately. This minute. Or the child will be scarred for life.

'Mam, you're soooooo mean! All my friends have this. All of them. I'm the only one who doesn't. I *hate* you.'

And naturally this guilt-tripping nightmare for parents is fully exploited by the cosmetics industry too. Get them young and you'll get them forever, goes the thinking. Irish people are notoriously brand loyal.

So you can see why the cosmetic companies are targeting a younger and younger consumer — it's good sense for them. And if you're a tween, it's good for you too: you're getting better products. And getting your parents to pay for them. As Mr Burns from *The Simpsons* would say, 'Eeeexcellent.'

The only group it's not working for is parents. Pester power is insidious and will wring every spare drop of cash out of you quicker than one of the IMF's doom-laden budgets.

Oh dear.

SPF

Look out for moisturiser that has a good SPF in it too — at least SPF 15 for Ireland. Sun damage is the biggest cause of old, tired, wrinkly skin later in life and if you're clued in about your products now, you'll stay younger and fresher looking forever.* There will be no need to totally avoid sunlight altogether — they go a bit too far with their anti-ageing regime in *Twilight*, don't they?

*May be a slight exaggeration.

Recommendations

Shop Smart: L'Oréal Paris Perfect Clean Foaming Gel Wash €

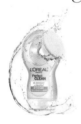

This is a foaming face wash with a secret weapon — the Scrublet, which gently exfoliates, leading to softer skin and clearer pores. Stick it to your shower wall to remind yourself to use it in the morning — genius!

Garnier Pure Active Exfo-Brusher Wash €

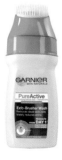

Removes dead skin cells and visibly reduces shine for the be-blackheaded amongst us. The 2 per cent salicylic acid in this formula shifts flaky, dead skin and really does reveal a new, smooth, lovely layer beneath. It also promises to fade those horrible marks and blemishes caused by spots. The nifty thing about this product is that the cap twists open to release the gel and then shuts to facilitate mess-free buffing with its 170 soft flexi-bristles.

Neutrogena Multi-Defence €

Designed to protect skin against UV rays and dehydration, these products are multitasking wonders that battle all sorts of environmental aggressors. Skin is shielded from cold, heat, wind, pollution and smoke at really affordable prices – everything's under a tenner. Particularly good for twenty-somethings upwards, there are different products for combination, normal, dry and sensitive skin.

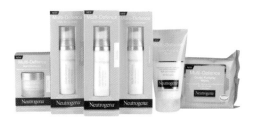

Origins Zero Oil €€€

The Origins Zero Oil range is packed with kick-ass cleansing ingredients like salicylic acid and saw palmetto. The gel wash smells refreshingly minty and works like Vichy Normaderm on steroids.

If you have a fecker of a time with spots and blackheads, Zero Oil is for you. This range is formulated to tackle oily and acne-prone skin and the foaming cleanser unclogs pores, reduces shine and controls oil during the day. Because it's Origins, it's full of natural ingredients, free from many chemical nasties and isn't tested on animals.

Dermalogica Clean Start Kit €€€

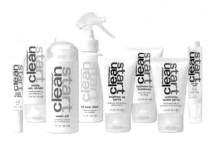

All of Dermalogica's ranges were developed for young skin and almost any of their products will suit teen and twenty-something skin depending on type. It was only when their customer base grew up and entered their thirties and forties that they developed the Age Smart range for older skin.

Segmenting their consumer groups this way worked, so now Dermalogica have specifically targeted the tween and teenage groups with Clean Start. Marketing ploy or not, it's still a pretty good range with eight products designed to take you through morning cleansing right through to bedtime.

The Wash Off cleanser is a particular winner. Smelling fresh and zesty, it's a good way to dip your toes into the range. And don't mind Dermalogica and all their guff about having to be prescribed products by a salon beautician. You can just go online and buy the range from loads of online shops – and it will be cheaper too.

Clarins Daily Energizer Range for Young Skin €€

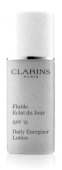

We're moving into premium brand territory with this range, but the prices in the Daily Energizer line are surprisingly good for such a high-end brand. There are five products, including a foaming cleanser gel and a good gel moisturiser that won't clog pores.

The cleanser contains moringa extract to help neutralise the effects of pollution and it leaves skin fresh and clear. This is nice skincare from a trusted brand and we'll doubtless see other brands following suit and bringing out young skin ranges.

Cult Product: Vichy Normaderm €€

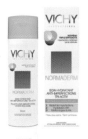

The entire Vichy Normaderm range is an absolute winner for hormone-ravaged teenage and twenty-something skin. From their oil-free moisturisers, night creams, super-effective spot cream and classic gel cleanser, this bright green range from Vichy is one that everybody loves. It's effective, it works brilliantly and once you've tried Normaderm you'll be a convert for life. If you suffer from congested skin you'll be thanking us forever for pointing you towards Normaderm.

Use Proper Cleanser

Get into the habit now of using proper cleanser to take your make-up off. Irish women love make-up wipes and the fact that they're our bestselling, er, 'cleanser' should make the nation hang its head in shame. Don't use them. They're crap and they don't cleanse down into your pores. Using a good foaming or gel cleanser instead will go a long way towards giving you great skin.

Beaut.ienomics:
Go for Good
Supermarket Brands

There's really no need to go for expensive products – you just need good, effective skincare that suits your skin and your pocket. The supermarkets and big chemists do great offers on this category of skincare – the best offers to go for here are 50 per cent (or more) extra free, buy one get one free (BOGOF) and buy three get cheapest free (this means you can get a cleanser, moisturiser and another product thrown in for nothing).

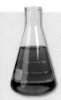

Read the Ingredients

● Salicylic Acid

An all-round wonder ingredient, this not only exfoliates skin but has also been proven to actually penetrate into whiteheads and blackheads and clean them out. It heals blemishes and makes skin smoother. Brilliant for any skin prone to clogging and especially good for young skin.

● Alcohol

Avoid like the plague. It's far too harsh and drying for skin that's erupting and breaking out and can cause even more skin hassles.

● Lanolin

A major cause of clogging and face cheese (a disgusting term used by Kirstie to describe gunk in the pores like blackheads/whiteheads or any other yucky stuff).

● Isopropyl Myristate

This can be used as an alternative to oil and may be used in some 'oil-free' products. Look out for it if you've got sensitive skin, as it can cause irritation.

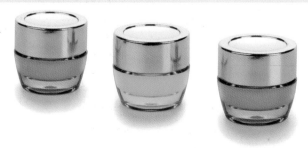

Anti-ageing

This is another category that has bucked the trend for recession spending. Instead of falling or merely holding steady as some categories are doing, our spending on anti-ageing products is actually rising — and this is the most expensive category of cosmetics out there.

The science can be baffling and some of the made-up terms are quite frankly ridiculous, so it's no wonder the average woman on the street doesn't know what's good or just hype any more. But the good news is that we do. We've sat through the seminars, we've read all the information and tested the products. The ones that we're recommending here are the best ones out there right now.

Beaut.ienomics: Pick Anti-Ageing Products with Clinical Trials to Back Them Up

Bravo to Boots for bringing their commitment to independent clinical trials and testing into sharp focus for consumers when they made such big waves with their Protect & Perfect products, but what you might not know is that lots of other mid-priced mass brands do exactly the same. Vichy, RoC, La Roche-Posay and L'Oréal Paris have routinely conducted extensive testing for many years and ploughed huge sums and efforts into developing new technologies, better delivery systems and improved ingredients. That means their products are well researched, tested and formulated and they're all decently priced too.

Recommendations

Shop Smart: Aldi Lacura Face Care Double Lift Regeneration Cream €

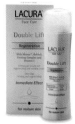

With its two colour-stripe it looks a bit like a tube of Aquafresh, but don't let that put you off. Ingredients like retinol to stimulate collagen production plus peptides and vitamin E add up to a very good combination of ingredients at a fraction of the price you will normally pay for a cream of this quality.

Shop Smart: L'Oréal Paris Youth Code Rejuvenating Anti-Wrinkle Day Cream €€€

Lots and lots of science here based on good results from clinical trials to prove it works means that this is a fantastic supermarket anti-ageing line. In a nutshell, skin is protected from stress and is able to recover from aggro (like nasty weather) more quickly, which keeps it looking good for longer.

Shop Smart: Garnier Vital Restore €€

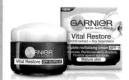

Well priced and effective, Vital Restore is targeted at fifty-plus skin, which has its own specific concerns: it can get drier than the Sahara, pick up age spots and sometimes seems to lose firmness by the day. This is why this skin type needs ultra-hydrating and firming ingredients that will also work to prevent further discolouration of the skin. The Vital Restore range includes day cream (SPF 15), night cream, eye cream and serum, all containing orchid extract and soy bio-protein to effectively firm and hydrate. The pretty pink glass jars will be welcome on any dressing table.

No7 Protect & Perfect Intense Day Cream SPF15 €€€

We're really liking the belt and braces approach to anti-ageing in this day cream. It has all the proven anti-ageing benefits of the Boots sell-out Protect & Perfect range plus broad spectrum sun protection to protect against future damage. It doesn't make any sense not to have a pot of this cream in your arsenal.

Vichy LiftActiv Retinol HA €€€€

This cream from Vichy proudly proclaims that it contains Retinol-A and hyaluronic acid. In addition, it's been clinically trialled and tested. Be careful with the applicator yoke though, as it has a tendency to squirt out a bit too much product. Apart from that, top marks for this – the day cream has an SPF of 18 and the night cream is fab too.

Nuxe Nuxuriance Anti-ageing Range €€€€€

The name is like a cross between luxurious and radiance and it's absolutely choc-a-block with ingredients to pep up tired skin. Hyaluronic acid of natural origin plumps and adds moisture. Caffeine brightens and perks up dull skin, making it a real treat.

Marks & Spencer Advanced Formula Peptides Firm & Lift Beauty Balm €€

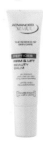

Reduce lines and wrinkles plus firm and smooth skin in just four weeks, says Marks & Spencer, who conducted good consumer trials on this balm. The magic ingredients are hexapeptides, which can plump out skin, and that alone has the effect of smoothing wrinkles up and out. There's also Siberian ginseng, which helps lift and tighten. It's a cheap and effective product with great ingredients – we love it.

RoC Sublime Energy €€€€

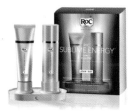

It may look messy and the first step is a siliconey balm with a gucky grey colour, but boy is it amazing. Skin cells communicate with each other to trigger the anti-ageing process and this results in more lovely elastin and collagen plumping up your skin. Ground-breaking science stuff here for a really decent price.

Trilogy CoQ10 Booster Serum €€€€

Strictly speaking this should go in the serum section, but as it's so targeted towards anti-ageing we let it sneak in here. This fantastic natural gloop contains CoQ10, tamanu and essential oils to nourish skin. Like a drink for skin that is quickly absorbed, it really does refresh and soften.

Lancôme Génefique €€€€€+

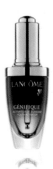

Lancôme Génefique – can I actually just say here that I love you. You were marketed as the best thing since sliced bread and, er, you *are* the best thing since sliced bread. Initially we were sceptical of the hype overload and the Youth Activator (the serum) doesn't suit everyone. It's the night and day creams that get a huge thumbs up – fantastically luxurious and delicious, they are well worth treating yourself to.

Prevage €€€€€+

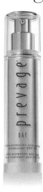

You may need a science degree to get to grips with the reasons why Prevage is so brilliant, but not to worry, we've checked it all out for you. Packed with antioxidants, including a new breed of super-antioxidant called Idebenone, the magic formulas protect skin against further damage and repair the look of what has already occurred, making short work of age spots, dull skin and the appearance of lines. High-performance, luxury skincare at its best. We think the song 'Nobody Does It Better' should be sung about Prevage. That's how much we love it.

Kiehl's Midnight Recovery Concentrate €€€€€

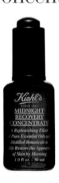

Two or three drops of this paraben-free botanical and essential oil-based serum does the trick while you get your zeds. Designed to replenish the lipids in the skin and keep it healthy – which is basically what keeps the skin's barrier intact – it's a clear, light fluid that's remarkably non-oily considering it contains loads of botanical and essential oils. Squalene, evening primrose, coriander and rosehip seed oils are the powerhouses here, dosing the skin with omegas 3, 6 and 9 and providing hydration and elasticity.

Estée Lauder Time Zone €€€€€

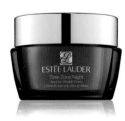

Not one but three hyaluronic technologies are combined here to make a super-duper line-busting anti-wrinkle range. Wrinkles are plumped up and sort of filled in to make everything look younger and fresher. The night cream is particularly yum in this range and will make your skin feel gorgeous when you wake up.

Cult Product: StriVectin SD Intensive Concentrate for Stretch Marks and Wrinkles €€€€€

A new, reformulated and better version of the original stretch mark cream, this also performs excellently on facial wrinkles, has extra peptides and boasts a texture akin to butter. The big size means you can use it on face and body: using the same product to zap arse marks and facial grooves has to be one of the most brilliant things ever.

Beaut.ienomics: Let Them Eat Peptides

As we mentioned earlier, anti-ageing is one of the few categories that is bucking the downward trend in cosmetics spending. Irish women are downsizing in other areas of spending – they would prefer to buy own brand groceries and do their weekly shop in Aldi or Lidl rather than give up their Chanel or Elemis wrinkle creams. These creams make women feel better about themselves, they make them look better and there's no way they're giving them up. No way.

Invest in Your Face

If you are really concerned about your skin and want to keep it looking young for as long as possible, think about visiting a dermatologist. They will assess your skin, determine the amount of sun damage you've got and recommend the best way to look after it. They will also have access to all the Botox, Fraxel, Restylane, fillers and other injectibles out there, but be warned that this is an expensive road to go down. Still, nothing works as well as these types of treatments and if you'd prefer to invest in your face rather than the stock market, then go for it. The stock market's not such a great bet right now anyway!

Read the Ingredients

Here are three great anti-ageing ingredients to look out for.

Peptides

Peptides are a huge buzzword at the moment, largely because of their potential in skincare. As we get older, skin stops manufacturing collagen and applying peptides (a part of the collagen protein) will hopefully trick skin into making some more and keeping it younger looking. Peptides can also attach to copper molecules and copper is great for keeping skin firm and regenerating it.

Retinol

Vitamin A derived from animal sources is known as retinol. Skin scientists and dermatologists tip the nod to vitamin A as one of the few beauty ingredients that's proven to actually turn back time on the ageing process. Even better is the fact that there are loads of products on the market — some at really reasonable prices — that use the retinol form of the ingredient too.

Hyaluronic Acid

Think of this as a moisture attracter, as it works a bit like a sponge, capable of holding many times its own weight in water. If you see this ingredient on a label it's a dead cert that it's going to deeply moisturise and plump up skin, lines, wrinkles and all. A real star ingredient, brilliant for both dry and ageing skin.

Just bear in mind that even though an ingredient label may list one of these wonders, it might be in a very small quantity indeed — you can often tell that by how far down a list of ingredients it appears. So watch out and don't believe label hype alone — go on recommendations too.

Beaut.ienomics:
Six Ways to Look Instantly Younger on the Cheap

Ever noticed on shows like *Ten Years Younger* that it's the hair, make-up and clothes that make most of the difference? Without even cracking open a costly bottle of pentapeptide-rich elixir, there are lots of things you can do to make yourself look instantly younger, and best of all, most of them are really cheap.

● Pluck Your Eyebrows

Heavy brows and long straggly bits are doing you no favours and will add years to your face. Invest in a good tweezers like a slanted Tweezerman (you only have to do it once), get your eyebrows shaped professionally and keep them that way. If you head to an Estée Lauder Brow Bar they will do a fantastic job on your brows and the money it costs is redeemable against purchase of cosmetics — a really good deal.

● Update Your Make-up

Yes, that make-up may have looked gorgeous 20 years ago, but if you're still using the exact same colours and foundation, chances are that the products don't suit you any more. Go to one of the lovely ladies at the make-up counters in your nearest department store or big chemist and tell them you're interested in updating your look. Keep an open mind and see what they recommend — and then get them to try it out on you. It's always great to see what someone else recommends and it can be a real eye opener.

Rethink Your Hairdo

It's so easy to get caught in a hair rut. Your cut and colour could be adding years to you. Get a good consultation to update the style and consider going a little lighter colourwise and possibly changing your style. Despite folk wisdom, women can and do look great with long hair when they're over 40.

Halve Your Salon Colour Visits

It costs an absolute blimmin fortune to get those roots touched up every six weeks, doesn't it? A lot of people are touching up their colour themselves with root kits (look at Clairol's Root Touch-Up for one to try) and saving themselves a lot of cash. Taking only 10 minutes and a really small spend compared with a salon visit, it's certainly a big money saver.

Paint Your Nails Yourself

Don't bother going for manicures – paint your nails yourself and ditch the French manicure, which is pretty ageing all on its own and is out of fashion at the moment. As nails are so on trend, a really quick and cheap way to update your look is to buy a shade of polish that's making beauty headlines. Choose a more chic version of the colours that are in and look at greige, nudes and beiges, as they tend to flatter and elongate the fingers. And you can have fun with nails – try matching them to your handbag or shoes. Go forth and paint!

Whiten Your Teeth

Yellowing teeth are yet another tell-tale sign of ageing, but luckily this is another thing that's easily and cheaply remedied. Don't bother with pricey laser-based whitening – the strips you get to put over your teeth often work just as well. Crest Whitestrips and Whizzer Whitening Strips are good ones to try.

Beaut.ienomics:
Four Smart Shopping Tips

Because the premium brands don't discount their products (when was the last time you saw a sale at the Chanel counter?), you have to be clever to save. If you've got a heavy anti-ageing product habit, there are four strategies that will save you money.

● Airport Shopping

With 25 to 40 per cent off cosmetics in the airport shops, you really can't afford not to stock up on your creams when you're passing through. We flew to Cork last year and stopped off at Airport Shopping on the way to the boarding gate to pick up a few bits and pieces. On the plane, we realised that the savings we'd made had paid for the flight.

● Pick Up Your Products Abroad

An extension of the airport shopping plan, really. If you're going on holiday (or have a sister-in-law who goes to New York every Christmas), get your skincare in another land – any land except Ireland, which is ridiculously expensive for everything. You'll save a fortune.

● Go Online

Think about it. No bricks and mortar stores, no customer service staff to pay – of course online is cheaper. On top of discounted prices, you can bag quite a bargain with special offers and sales too. Shopping online is perfectly safe, so go forth and save.

● Don't Dismiss Own Brand

Don't be snobby about your products. Don't say, 'Oh, I would only use Sisley' and dismiss other brands out of hand. Own brand manufacturers spend their lives copying premium cosmetics and presenting them to you at a fraction of the price. Get out of that brand loyal mindset and you'll save a lot of money.

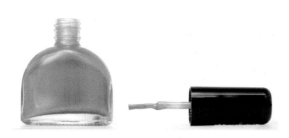

Sensitive Skin

Did you know that sensitive skin is actually a dermatological condition? It is, and it's very common here thanks to our pale, thin Irish skin. We're a particularly reactive population and one that's also prone to conditions like rosacea, eczema and psoriasis. As a result, it's a bit of a holy grail search to hunt down good, reliable ranges for sensitive skin.

And it's not just us gals who need them: men suffer terribly from skin issues too and can use all of the ranges mentioned here. They don't need to buy a fancy 'man brand' – which will be loaded with manly scent and in black/navy packaging – but can stick to these simple fragrance-free products too. They won't know themselves.

Sensitive and reactive skins are very difficult to give blanket recommendations for though, as it is almost impossible to ensure that a particular ingredient won't react with your particular skin monster. If you're suffering from spots, acne or have teenage skin issues, then check out our section on Young Skin (pp. 2–8).

Fragrance Watch

Stand-out brands we rate for sensitive skin are La Roche-Posay, Trilogy, Seavite and Avène and they've all worked hard to remove the nasties from their sensitive ranges. Do go carefully even so, especially if scent is listed in the ingredients. Fragrance is a big cause of reaction in sensitive skin, so watch out for this even if a product is targeted at your skin type.

Recommendations

Shop Smart: Cetaphil €€

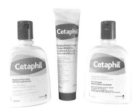

This bargaintastic range is brilliant for the sensitive among us. Big bottles of cleanser, moisturiser and body lotion seem to get on well with almost everyone and are definitely worth trying. The stand-out product is the cleanser: it's non-drying and takes make-up off really well (a major gripe with most sensitive skin cleansers is that they don't remove make-up properly), either with or without water. So if you react to everything, including water, this might well work for you.

Shop Smart: Lidl Cien Moisturiser for Sensitive Skin €

Packed full of skin-soothing ingredients like aloe vera, this was definitely a surprise find for us. It is rated by the most sensitive skinned gals (who were normally fans of pricier brands) who found that it calmed and nourished and, best of all, didn't cause any reaction.

Trilogy Sensitive Skin €€€

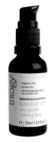

While the entire Trilogy range is a good bet for reactive types, the Sensitive Skin line goes one better and is really mild and gentle. Try Trilogy Very Gentle Cleansing Cream if you can't take off make-up without stinging the face off yourself. It's a fragrance-free, water-based cleansing cream packed with pure plant oils, including camellia and chamomile, which calm and soothe. This should remove your eye make-up without leaving you staggering around the bathroom desperately groping for a towel to blot your eyes with. Use the Very Gentle Calming Fluid alone or as a serum before your moisturiser. It's a good product which can bring an extra layer of hydration to your routine.

Clinique Redness Solutions Instant Relief Mineral Powder €€€€

A sort of cross between skincare and make-up, this hybrid fairy dust will calm down the most rosy of faces. The yellow colour neutralises flushes and blushes: it disguises high colour and actually calms it too. As it's a mineral powder, it can be drying, so if you don't get on wonderfully well with minerals, use this just where you need it. For use after your cleanse and moisturise steps, it can be applied under or over make-up, used on its own or with foundation.

Eucerin €€

It might not be the sexiest, but Eucerin is a good affordable bet for those with sensitivities or suffering from atopic or extremely dry skin. Cleansers, moisturisers, eye creams and lots more are on offer.

Guaranteed Irish: Elave €

Made in Ireland, Elave products can be used by those prone to eczema, sensitivity, dermatitis, rosacea and psoriasis. The Elave Dermatological Range is very well priced and packed full of products for face and body that contain only the safest non-reactive ingredients.

La Roche-Posay €€

One of the best all-round sensitive skincare lines, we highly rate this French brand for its excellent products. Scent free, kind and caring, it's also really affordable.

Cult Product: Avène €€€

Beloved of beauty editors and those in the know for its efficacy, Avène is a French brand that we haven't seen much of in Ireland until recently. Happily, it's now much more widely available in stockists near you. These unscented products really take care of skin: extremely dry, irritated, acne-prone, super-sensitive and redness are all problems that Avène has ranges for. There are also products for anti-ageing and suncare, cleanser for oily, blemish-prone skin as well as one of the brand's star products, its Eau Thermale spritz, which gives offerings from Evian, Vichy and La Roche-Posay a run for their money.

Tip Baby Knows Best

If you find you can't tolerate anything from the beauty counter, then this could be one instance where baby knows best. Infant skincare products have to be very specifically formulated to take into account the fact that babies have such delicate skins and little barrier function. Products aimed at tots are typically very kind and gentle and could work well for you, too.

Beaut.ienomics: Aqueous Cream

One of the best – and most Beaut.ienomical – products we've ever come across for sensitive and reactive skin types is plain old aqueous cream. You can buy it in any chemist the land over, it costs half nothing and can be called into play for a variety of uses, including cleansing and washing very delicate skin.

Cleansers

W e're always banging on about this, but cleansing really is the cornerstone of your beauty routine. It removes grunge, grime and the dirt of the day, whips off dead skin cells and gives your skin a clean canvas on which to apply serum and moisturiser. Daily cleansing with products that suit your skin will be one of the best beauty habits you can ever take up.

There are a plethora of new cleansing products on the market and innovations like glycolic and salicylic acids are used to good effect in many cleansers, but the cult products are as good as ever. This is great, as a super-pricey cleanser is usually copied by mass market brands – hot cloth cleansers are a case in point. We've tried out a lot of cleansers on your behalf – read on and see what we rate.

Beaut.ienomics: Stick with the Range That Suits You

If you have a budget skincare range that you get on well with, chances are that the cleanser in that line will suit you down to the ground. There's no need to pay over the odds if you've got normal skin either: if you're getting on well with Nivea or L'Oréal Paris, then stick with them for cleanser. The products in this section are recommended for those who want to try something a bit different and see what all the cleansing fuss is about.

Wipes – Still the Work of Satan

Yes, face wipes are still the work of Beelzebub himself and should be ejected forthwith to the bowels of hell. Or the bin – whichever is nearest. Yes, we know you like to use them because they're quick, but they're just not kind to your skin and they won't do you any favours in the long run. Seriously, ditch the wipes and be amazed at how much better your skin can look.

Try Oil

Oils are kind of like our cosmetic crack: we adore 'em for hair and skin and they make brilliant cleansers too. We're just not into the fuss of cream and milk cleansers and mounds of dirty tissues and cotton pads, and you won't be either when you've made the leap to an oil or a balm. They literally take every scrap of make-up off in seconds and leave skin feeling clean and calm, with none of the tightness often associated with gel cleansers.

Recommendations

Soap & Glory Fab Pore Hot Cloth Cleanser €€

Fans of Liz Earle's famous Cleanse & Polish Hot Cloth Cleanser will like this: it's creamy and deliciously scented. When used with a hot muslin cloth, it really cleanses skin and removes all traces of make-up.

MAC Cleanse Off Oil €€€

Cleansing oils are a firm favourite for their sheer efficacy, power-packed performance and ease of use. MAC's Cleanse Off Oil is well-priced, we reckon, as one or two pumps is enough to cleanse skin of even the most heavy-duty slap, so a little goes a long way.

Eve Lom Morning Time €€€€

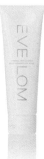

With spices like cinnamon, this cleanser smells like a Christmas cake. The balm turns into an oil when it warms up on your skin, making it easy to use. Gentle papaya extract exfoliates and you can feel a slightly rough texture declogging your pores. Despite the name, it's not just for morning, but it's not great at taking off make-up. Better kept for a second cleanse after the make-up has been washed down the drain.

Body Shop Nutriganics Softening Cleansing Gel €€

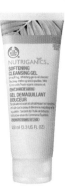

One of the new breed of gel-to-oil cleansers, this is a lovely product to use. It's nicely scented, can be massaged into skin and removed with warm water. You can rinse it off with your fingers, but we like to give it an extra bit of help by removing it with a muslin cloth. What's also fab about this is it's EcoCert certified, so those who like to use organic and natural skincare can rest easy.

REN ClearCalm 3 Anti-Blemish Clay Cleanser €€€

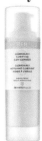

This antibacterial cleanser works deep into the pores of problem skin, using clay to draw out impurities and natural goodies like manuka honey to calm and sooth blemishes. If you like Dermalogica's Dermal Clay Cleanser, then you'll get on well with this.

Elemis Melting Cleansing Gel €€€

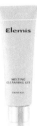

The gel-to-oil formula used here is a bit like the cult Clarins Pure Melt Cleansing Gel. It smells yum – citrusy and just all-round super-sniffable. Effective at removing make-up and leaving skin super soft, this is a really good cleanser. And yes, it is pricey, but it *is* Elemis, and you only use a tiny bit so it goes a long way.

Tesco Vitamin E Cleanser €

Tesco Vitamin E Cleanser is the bestselling cleanser in Tesco! Yep, it outsells absolutely everything. We suspect the reason is because it's so cheap and not because it's completely brilliant at what it does.

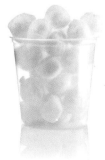

Muslin Cloths

We love, love, love muslin cloths because they really add an extra aspect to your cleansing routine. Slightly scrubby, you can use a cloth wrung out in hot water to remove an oil, balm or even a milk cleanser. You get a little exfoliation each time you use your cloth, so it helps to cut down on using a separate exfoliator. In fact, we find we rarely need to use our beloved Origins Modern Friction any more.

Woolite Your Muslin Cloths

Muslin cloths go manky, it's true. But you don't have to throw them out because you can give them a new lease on life. We boil ours up in a saucepan with a slug of Woolite, throw them in a hot wash and they come up (almost) as good as new.

Eye Make-up Remover

Recommendations

Johnson's Daily Essentials Gentle Eye Make-up Remover €

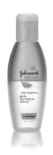

Sure, you can spend a lot of cash on a pricier eye make-up remover, but this dual-phase one from Johnson's is just as good as a much more expensive one from Lancôme or Clinique. Shake it together, lash some on a cotton pad and watch your shadow and mascara dissolve. But if you like fancy brands, see what we rate below.

Cult Product: Lancôme Bi-Facil €€€

Give this a shake to mix both liquids in the bottle and then squoosh a dollop onto a cleansing pad. While it says it's non-oily, feck that, it *is* oily, and that's what makes it so good at getting all sorts of guck off your eyes. Glitter, waterproof mascara, smoky eyes, primer and pigment don't stand a chance. A good sample size of this is often included in Lancôme Gift Time – try it out then and you'll be hooked.

Exfoliators

Origins Modern Friction €€€€€

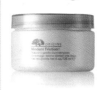

An oldie but such a goodie: this is pricey initially but lasts and lasts – oh, and it lasts some more. Containing rice grains, it gently polishes skin and is really good for getting hormonal spotty breakouts back under control and skin looking fresh and clean again.

La Roche-Posay Physiological Ultra-Fine Scrub €€

This is a really nice scrub. You can feel it working but it doesn't leave skin feeling rubbed raw or irritated. And because it's got nicely medicinal packaging, men like using it too.

Benefit Refined Finish Facial Polish €€€

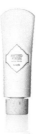

This is a deliciously fresh facial polish that uses micro beads and clay to gently slough off dead skin cells and refine pores. Use a couple of times a week after your cleanser (use the Benefit Foamingly Clean Facial Wash if you like, it's also good). The packaging is pleasingly tactile, and with their chunky cork lookalike lid, this range looks so pretty. Check out the Young Skin section (pp. 2–8) for lots more cleanser recommendations.

A Softer Scrub

If your face scrub is too, well, scrubby, then mix it with a little cream or milk cleanser to make it less abrasive. *Et voilà*! A kinder, gentler product that'll still buff your skin nicely.

Serums

The elixir of the skincare gods, serum is packed full of active ingredients and that's what makes it so potent and good for the skin. Unfortunately, that's also the reason why it can be so pricey. Happily, though, we're now seeing mid-priced brands like Olay, L'Oréal Paris and Vichy offering really decent alternatives at affordable prices.

Serum FAQs

So, um, what exactly is a serum?

A serum is a first-step product that usually contains a concentrated dose of good-for-skin ingredients such as antioxidants, collagen, peptides, retinyl palmitate (a form of retinol) and hyaluronic acid. They're designed to be used as part of your routine as a booster and to deliver a shot of extra nutrients to the skin.

Do I need one?

Generally best for those who've already begun to explore the whole sphere of anti-ageing products, you probably won't need to add a serum until you're in your thirties. If you're starting to notice lines, wrinkles, pigmentation spots and dull, dry skin, then you should definitely think about it. If you're younger and find you can't keep moisture in your skin, a hydrating serum could boost your moisture levels.

Does it replace my moisturiser?

No, definitely not. You use serum before your moisturiser as an extra step and then carry on as normal.

A serum is not the second coming of Christ

Lots of rubbish abounds in press releases and marketing materials from brands when they launch a new serum. You can expect to be blinded by science and subjected to 'miracle this' and 'Botox in a bottle' that as well as more baffling percentages than you can shake a stick at.

We're all for products that work, but we often wish brands would quit it with over-claiming, because it just alienates us as beauty consumers. All too often, claims are hyperbole-filled claptrap: nothing can give the effect of Botox except, er, Botox. And as for miracle? Ah here, we're talking about a skincare product, not the second coming of Christ. Do expect some results like a lessening of fine lines and an improvement in skin tone and texture, but don't be expecting a whole new face because you will be disappointed.

Recommendations

L'Oréal Paris Youth Code Serum Intense €€€

Part of the brilliant Youth Code range, this anti-ageing serum has lots of serious science to back it up. It's a light serum that feels nice to use and is offered in tandem with day, night and eye creams, so if you find you like it, you can indulge in the whole shebang.

Clinique Even Better Clinical Dark Spot Corrector €€€€€

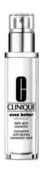

With great results to back the claims made by Clinique for this product, it is definitely worth taking a look if you have mild pigmentation issues. This has a cumulative effect – the longer you use it, the better the results. It works by gently exfoliating off the patchy areas of pigmentation and has been enjoying a lot of success since it launched. Once you don't expect instant results, you won't be disappointed – you need to give this one a chance.

Marks & Spencer Advanced Formula Peptides Ultimate Serum €€

As this has quite a dry texture, we think it's a good bet for someone with normal-to-combination skin who is looking for some extra nourishment, plumping and firming of the skin.

Vichy LiftActiv CxP Total Day Serum €€€€

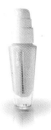

This anti-ager stimulates collagen production, leading to an increase in skin firmness. Sinks in well and has some cosmetic trickery in there in the form of mother of pearl extract, which immediately adds a glow to the skin. Good science, price and easy availability are also big pluses in its favour.

Guaranteed Irish: Kinvara Rejuvenate Rosehip Face Serum €€€

Formulated in the West of the country for our typical Irish skin – reactive, sensitive and downright sick of harsh weather, this is soothing, restoring and packed full of antioxidants. We think this is a terrific serum that's all-natural, organic and smells absolutely delicious.

Kiehl's Açaí Damage-Repairing Serum €€€€€

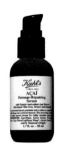

Açaí is where it's at these days. Pronounced ah-sigh-ee, this little wonder fruit is packed full of antioxidants and is also rich in essential fatty acids. That means it's excellent for repair and nourishment – antioxidants help to battle the free radicals responsible for skin ageing and essential fatty acids are good at adding moisture to the skin and therefore plumping it up, which helps to iron out any crinkles.

No7 Protect & Perfect Beauty Serum €€€

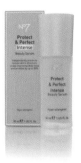

This is the one that all the fuss was about. Clinical trials proved that it worked and we went nuts to get our hands on it as a result. Its ability to improve skin is down to the fact it includes a form of easily tolerated retinol, which is a proven anti-ager. Plus it's got a nice silky feel and forms a good base for make-up.

Cult Product: Estée Lauder Advanced Night Repair Synchronized Recovery Complex €€€€€

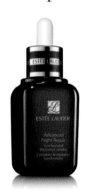

Phew! The name is a bit of a mouthful, but asking for 'the new Night Repair' at the Estée Lauder counter will do the trick. This orange gloop is as good as it gets. It wins all the awards and praise for a reason – it really does make skin look better. The new version is even more sci-fi and like the name says is designed for use at night.

Facial Oils

Facial oils are a scrumptious addition to any beauty routine. In the cold, harsh weather of winter their moisturising capabilities can literally stop your face from collapsing into a heap of dust like the Wicked Witch of the West. We love oils even more than we love serums, which is saying a lot. They're brilliant.

Facial Oil FAQs

We know it's a bit confusing if you're a novice. Are we talking about cooking oil or vegetable oil? No! Facial oils are created from plant and botanical oils and are full of lovely fatty acids and nourishing goodies. Here are some more things you need to know.

● Who are they good for?

Plant-based oils are particularly excellent for those with dry skin or who are experiencing the first signs of ageing, such as fine lines, which are often just dehydration in the skin. Oils also have what's known as a normalising effect and can be used to treat like with like. In other words, don't ignore them if you have oily skin.

● What should I look for?

Most good facial oils will contain a blend of different plant, flower and seed oils to deliver an optimum effect. Rose or rosehip oil is very nourishing and great at fighting off the ageing process, as is argan oil. Avocado, almond, hemp seed, chamomile and lavender are also often used.

Water Makes Oil Go Further

Apply oil to damp skin: it absorbs better because the water will draw the oil into the skin. You use less and a bottle lasts longer, saving you money.

Do I use oil instead of my moisturiser?

Oil *is* moisturiser, it's just not in a cream or emulsion format, so treat it as you would your regular product. So if you use a moisturiser daily, then use your oil daily. If you find that you don't need the richness of an oil every day, then use it as a treatment a couple of times a week.

Recommendations

Shop Smart: Marks & Spencer Formula Age Repair Phytoceramide Treatment Oil €€

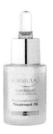

We reckon this is best for those with normal-to-combination skin, as it doesn't pack quite enough of a punch for anyone particularly Kalahari-complexioned. For the small outlay it's got some good ingredients in the form of essential oil of mandarin, apricot, sunflower and soya oils as well as sweet almond and rosehip.

Trilogy Rosehip Oil €€

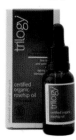

Fast approaching cult product status, this is one little bottle of magic you absolutely have to try. Unscented, it doesn't smell fabulous, but you won't care once you see what fab things it does for your face. This nourishing potion is clinically proven to reduce the signs of ageing and it can be used on stretch marks too. Love.

Liz Earle Superskin Concentrate €€€

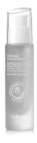

Oh lordy lord, how we love this (and its accompanying moisture cream). It's strongly scented with botanical oils and is packed full of goodies like cranberry and argan oils, which skin absolutely adores. This helps keep winter-ravaged skin on an even keel and is great for battling dehydration.

Naturelle d'Argan Pure Argan Elixir €€

Argan oil is a good ingredient to use if you're concerned about ageing and keeping skin in great nick. Many facial oils use it as part of their ingredients, but Naturelle d'Argan Pure Argan Elixir uses it solo to reap maximum benefits. It's an ingredient that's got a good beauty provenance and which is lauded for its nourishing and hydrating abilities.

Bobbi Brown Extra Face Oil €€€€€

Not a lot of people seem to know about this oil, which is a shame as it's darned good. Extra Face Oil is a drink for very thirsty skin and contains lots of oils like sesame, sweet almond, olive and jojoba as well as vitamin E. It's also a really good bet for mature complexions.

Eve Taylor Pre-Blended Facial Oil €€

This lovely oil comes in different varieties so you can really tailor it to your skin type, including sebum prone. Bonuses here are a pump dispenser, which we like – other products can be pretty messy. The scent of these products is to die for and they are also really well priced. Definitely worth a look.

Cult Product: Clarins Blue Orchid Oil €€€€€

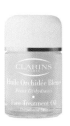

This smells yum, contains loads of nourishing goodies like orchid and hazelnut oils and is specifically designed to combat dehydration. Fret not if you don't answer to that particular description: there are also Clarins oils for dry/very dry and combination skins.

Beaut.ienomics: Green and Greedy

If there's one class of product that's bucking the downward spiral of recession spending, it's natural and organic products.

Natural and organic make-up and skincare used to be a niche market and you could only buy such products in specialised beardy weirdy shops. Now, however, this trend has gone mainstream and almost every big brand has launched a 'natural' range to complement their existing product lines.

This hasn't happened because of kindness to the environment or concerns about your delicate skin. No, it's about money.

Consumer fears about chemicals in products, in food – everywhere, in fact – are at an all-time high and this fear is exploited and exacerbated by advertising. Cosmetic brands prey on this fear and the wholesale introduction of natural and organic ranges means they have a perfect solution to the problem they caused themselves. Clever, eh?

A premium is slapped on organic and natural ranges. They cost more, but because we're worried about the effect of chemicals, we buy them anyway.

So it may be natural and green, but the prices are obscene.

Moisturisers

If there is one product most of us honestly can't live without, it's good old-fashioned moisturiser. It keeps skin comfortable and hydrated and there is so much choice out there, you're sure to find the perfect one for you. If you're a bit boggled by the selection on the shelves though, never fear – have a read through this section and find out what really hit the spot for us this year. (Remember, if you've got specific concerns, check out the Anti-ageing (pp. 9–19), Young Skin (pp. 2–8) or Sensitive Skin (pp. 20–23) sections.)

Beaut.ienomics:
Try Before You Buy

Look out for free samples in magazines and always ask for samples when you buy a product – that way, you get to try another product in the range. It's always good to see if something suits you before you hand over the cash. Some brands are notoriously stingy with their trial sizes, but we like these for their commitment to sampling:

- Clarins
- Kiehl's
- L'Occitane
- La Roche-Posay
- Lancôme
- Vichy

Why has my moisturiser suddenly stopped working?

We're all subject to the vagaries of time (not to mention the weather and our hormones), so if you find that the lovely fluid emulsion that worked so well for you in your twenties is letting you down now that you're 31, then it's time to make a change to a thicker formulation.

Similarly, if the product you used in the summer is suddenly useless now that it's five below and you're in and out of cold and central heating all day long, it's time to bust a move to something new. Or perhaps you've just come off the Pill or are new to it? That too can affect skin and cause your tried-and-trusted products to lose their effectiveness.

Lifestyle factors can nearly always be blamed for a sudden shift in your skin, so if you've suddenly noticed that your holy grail cream isn't doing the trick, look back over the past couple of months of your life – have you been on medication, are you stressed, pregnant or are there any other external factors that may be the cause? In addition, skin changes after 30 and so should your products. If any of these situations rings a bell, then it's a classic case of 'it's not you, it's me' and time to move on to a new moisturiser.

Recommendations

Shop Smart: Nivea Visage Natural Beauty Radiance Boosting Moisturiser €

This is a lovely product that has some added rose-gold shimmery radiance particles included, so it gives skin a glow. If you're having a super-duper good skin day wear it solo, but you can of course layer foundation over the top. It moisturises well and those with normal-to-dry skin will like its nourishing ways.

Shop Smart: Johnson's Daily Essentials €

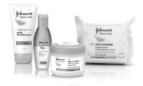

We've been trusting Johnson's since we were chislers and this is a good range of basic products, with day and night creams to suit every skin type. A great staple for every teen/twenty-something, especially as everything is priced at €5.

RoC Hydra+ 24Hr Comfort Nourishing Cream €€

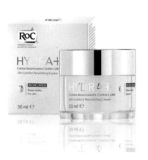

A great moisturiser from this French brand, who really know their stuff. This cream is targeted at the twenty- and thirty-somethings amongst us who have the whole work-drinks-club-fall-into-bed routine down to a fine art. What RoC is really saying is: you go have fun and we'll look after the moisturiser. Continuous hydration is the buzzword here. Sounds good to us and we really like this range.

Burt's Bees Radiance Day Creme €€€

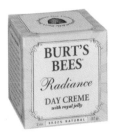

Burt's Bees looks like a cutesy wutesy line, but it's seriously good and should be taken seriously. Our readers rave about this skincare and really love the Radiance Day Creme. It's made with royal jelly, botanical oils and loads of other natural ingredients and will work with most skin types.

Benefit Triple Performing Facial Emulsion €€€

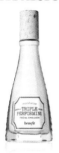

An oil-free moisturiser that's lightweight, smells fresh and provides SPF 15. Apply it after cleansing – even oily skin needs a drop of the right sort of hydration to keep it feeling soft and comfortable after cleansing. And the glass bottle is like something Betty Draper might have on her bedside table – very pretty indeed.

Vichy Normaderm Tri-Activ Anti-Imperfection Hydrating Care €€

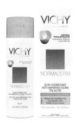

Perfect for oily skin, this triple-threat moisturiser promises to provide 24-hour continuous hydration while maintaining a matte finish and treating imperfections. Glycolic acid, salicylic acid and LHA (lipo-hydroxy acid) micro-exfoliate the skin's surface to target blemishes, blackheads and open pores and promote a smoother, more uniform complexion.

Avène Extremely Rich Compensating Cream €€€

For very dry and sensitive skin, this cream is very rich indeed and perfect for the ravages of winter. The only downside: we have diagnosed an increase in face cheese as a result of its use. We're not too bothered: we enjoy a joke and this is keeping those long-fought side-of-eye lines at bay.

L'Occitane Ultra Rich Face Cream €€€€

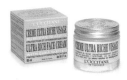

You practically have to fight this out of the pot, it's so thick, and is a great one to have on hand for very dry skin thanks to 25 per cent shea butter in the mix. If the scent isn't a deal-breaker (it can be a bit strong for some), you'll love this rich potion.

Darphin Hydraskin Essential All-Day Skin-Hydrating Emulsion €€€€

Although Darphin have the reputation of being one of the most expensive brands in the universe, they've started to come down to earth a bit with this range. The price is much better (think Estée Lauder instead of Crème de la Mer). This is still fancy though, using the technology of cacti (indeed) and other scrummy ingredients like shea butter. And the best bit? Well, they've put their sterling prices on a par with ours and for that we applaud them.

Cult Product: Clinique Superdefense SPF 25 Age Defense Moisturise €€€€

We like this moisturiser a lot. The consistency is great, it does the all-important sinking in quickly and efficiently and it provides a great base for make-up. It's also packed full of science – anti-ageing ingredients, antioxidants and SPFs. All good stuff and you can really trust this cream to put up the shields – keeping the moisture in and the bad guys (environmental aggressors, etc.) out.

Tip Remember to choose a moisturiser with at least an SPF of 15 if you aren't using a separate suncream.

Beaut.ienomics:
The Myth of the Irish Metrosexual

I don't mean to offend anyone here when I say that the average Irish male is totally Neanderthal when it comes to taking any care of his appearance. The painful scrape of a rusty razor over Sahara-dry skin is what's regarded as male grooming around these parts by the majority of men. Admitting to anything more soothing and beneficial to skin would be as socially shameful as donning a pink tutu and ordering a cosmo in the pub after the match.

It's a sad state of affairs in more ways than one. Male grooming was just taking off in Ireland as the Celtic Tiger roared and men in Ireland actually got over the slagging and started to use moisturiser. Women were the drivers of the demand for high-end products for men. An abundance of surplus income meant that women went out and bought the fancy ranges for their men, creating a boom. But when I say that they created a surge in the market, bear in mind that we were starting from a very low base. Very low.

But it was not to last. As the recession bit and disposable income shrank, this was the part of the shopping list that was the first to be ruthlessly cut from the budget. Women prioritised. Well, he didn't really appreciate it anyway, went the thinking, and I can't afford to buy his Lancôme and my Lancôme – so I choose mine. If he wants it, let him buy it for himself. But he hasn't been buying it for himself, so Irish men have just gone back to their weather-beaten ways. Most of them don't even remember this brief footnote in history or care about it either.

Hope lies with the new generation of urban Irish teens and twenty-somethings who have grown up with a healthy attitude to male grooming. Spending a little cash on skin and hair care products is second nature to them and they will continue with their face wash and moisturiser habit.

Ireland will just have to wait a bit longer for guyliner, manscara and Touche Éclat for men to take hold.

Eye Creams

Eye cream is probably the most mind-blowingly expensive beauty purchase on a ml by ml basis you'll make and there is lots of conflicting advice out there as to whether we actually need it or not. The answer is: if you feel you need it and it's doing your skin good, then go for it. The most important things that eye cream will do are to treat the sensitive skin around the eyes kindly, not weigh it down with heavy product and firm and hydrate. So without further ado, here are some creams that suit almost everyone.

Beaut.ienomics:
Beware of Overinflated Eye Cream Claims

Eye cream is expensive. Often eyewateringly expensive (excuse the pun). All sorts of magical claims are made for eye cream: that it will get rid of all your lines, wrinkles and crow's feet (it won't). All it can do is hydrate and soothe the skin under your eyes. Some of the most expensive creams claim to get rid of dark circles, but the simple fact is they can't and they won't. Darkness under the eyes is caused by lots of things that no cream can tackle, like tiredness, bad diet, genetics or a medical issue (for example, a kidney infection). If a cream proclaims it will 'lessen the appearance of dark circles', what that usually means is that it has some kind of light-reflecting ingredient in its formula and you'd be as well picking up a tube of under-eye concealer from Aldi and saving yourself about €100.

The Right Age for Eye Cream

Like most things in beautyland, there really are no rules. In general, you most likely don't need to start using eye cream any younger than your mid-twenties and most of us wait until we're into our thirties before it becomes a must-have. But if you'd like to use it earlier, go ahead – pick a nice light eye cream in the same range as your favourite moisturiser. Something with a gel formulation would be a good pick.

Recommendations

Shop Smart: Nivea Visage Q10PLUS Anti-Wrinkle Eye Cream €€

The Nivea Q10 range is a very good one and is excellent for the price. The science behind this eye cream (and the rest of the range) means that these products deliver, and the fact that they're bestsellers means that they're standing the test of time. A lovely, light, fresh eye cream.

Bobbi Brown Extra Eye Repair Cream €€€€€

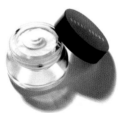

Light and very moisturising, it's been specially formulated to work well with make-up. Contains peptides, plant oils and other goodness to hydrate and diminish puffiness. In very cold weather this is a godsend and we lightly tap it into place at the sides of the eyes. Plus it comes in a pleasing chunky glass jar that looks only gorgeous.

Lancôme Rénergie Yeux Multiple Lift €€€€€+

Absolutely packed with lifting and brightening science, this lightweight eye cream has another trick up its sleeve: it contains a tinted illuminating treatment that works well with all skin tones and makes you look instantly fresher.

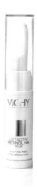

Vichy LiftActiv Retinol HA Total Wrinkle Care Eyes €€€

This is the heavy hitter to look for if you're concerned about deep lines around the eyes. Containing the proven anti-ageing ingredient retinol, it helps to take down those lines. Hydrating hyaluronic acid moisturises too.

Burt's Bees Radiance Eye Cream €€€

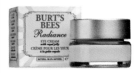

We're seeing a lot of love for this all-natural eye cream. Royal jelly is the star ingredient, helping to attract and keep moisture in the skin. A good choice if you don't want or need to move on to a specific anti-ageing eye cream.

Estée Lauder Advanced Night Repair Eye Recovery Complex €€€€€

Eagerly awaited, we don't know one single person who has used this eye cream and doesn't like it. Hyaluronic acid means that it attracts moisture and plumps up skin, while antioxidants fight off future damage.

Cult Product: Elizabeth Arden Ceramide Gold Ultra Lift and Strengthening Eye Capsules €€€€€

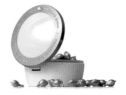

We love this box full of wonders, like little golden fishies. The serum inside the capsules spreads easily out over the eye area and just needs to be patted gently into place. It rehydrates and firms the under-eye area very quickly indeed – a couple of days and you'll notice a difference.

Beaut.ienomics:
Bonus Time

'Bonus time' or 'gift with purchase' is a perfect time to get to grips with a brand's newest eye cream. Our love for bonus time is well documented and we'll say it again: it's a great time to get to try products from a brand you'd never shell out the cash for.

Ask for a Sample

Before spending half your salary on a tiny pot of cream the size of a speck of dust, make sure it's actually good, that you like the texture and it doesn't sting the eyes off you. Ask one of the nice ladies at a department store counter for a sample. The next time you're replacing your moisturiser is a perfect time to put in a sample request. Tell the assistant you're interested in trying an eye cream from her range and chances are she'll give you great advice and a couple of packets of gloop to take home to try.

Puffy Eye Soother

Sometimes when you wake up in the morning you've got pronounced puffy bags under your eyes. Elevating your head a little more at night can help, as can keeping a teaspoon or two in the fridge. Take it out and press the rounded side gently against the lower eye. The cold metal will help to take down the puffiness. (Psst: this also works on hungover mornings when you look more Deputy Dawg than deadly.)

Lip Balms

The ultimate impulse buy, lip balms are small, portable and incredibly comforting and necessary in the type of weather we've been having over the last couple of winters. Winter air typically contains 30 per cent less moisture than warmer air, which makes it much more drying.

While any thick layer of salve would do the trick to act as a barrier against the elements (hence the enduring popularity of Vaseline), the lip balms listed here go far beyond the call of duty and add moisture and treatment benefits. If it's smelling delicious and intensely moisturising while keeping your lips soft and kissing ready you're after, these boyos will do it.

Lip Balm Addiction

No such thing. You might feel you need to keep applying lip balm if it's a product like Vaseline: all this does is shield your lips from the elements. The second it wears off, your lips are sore and chapped again and so you need to put some more on. It's a vicious cycle of lip balm application! This is why people think they're addicted. Choose a lip balm that actually treats the chapping and moisturises your lips and you'll soon find that you're not actually addicted at all.

Recommendations

Shop Smart: Vichy Aqualia Thermal Lip Balm €

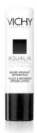

Super soft and smoothes everything out beautifully. Not too greasy, it's like a silky Chapstick, is suitable for sensitive skin and really helps to sort out tight, sore lips.

Burt's Bees Sun Protecting Lip Balm SPF 8 €

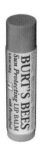

An incredibly popular all-natural, sweet-smelling and moisturising balm, this one ticks all the right boxes. It's important to protect lips from the sun, so the addition of an SPF is very smart.

Carmex €

Chapped lips quail at the sight of a tube of Carmex. It contains a blend of menthol, camphor and phenol to help heal chapped and sore lips and now comes in tasty fruity flavours.

Kiehl's Lip Balm #1 €€

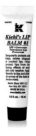

This is a clever product because it does two things: one, it's got petroleum jelly in there (yup, the same stuff as Vaseline), which acts as a barrier on the lips, and two, it's got lots of hydrating and nourishing ingredients that can hide behind that barrier and do your lips some good. It's pricey, but really well thought out.

Neutrogena Immediate Repair Lip Balm €

This is a man's lip balm. And by that we mean it's super strong and silent (lip balm doesn't tend to chat that much anyway). If you want a no nonsense product that's rich and nourishing, this is yer only man. Hey, if it can stand up to Arctic weather conditions, who are we to argue?

Crème de la Mer The Lip Balm €€€€€+

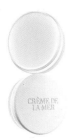

Super posh – why not treat yourself to a little of the Crème magic? We bought ours before the arse fell out of the economy and it's a really superb product. This is the littlest part of the range you can buy – just remember not to lose it because it does not have a little price!

Nivea SOS Lip Balm €

Calming, soothing and super cheap. This one gets lots of love, and if you lose it out of your coat pocket you won't feel too bad about it.

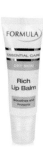

Marks & Spencer Formula Dry Skin Rich Lip Balm €

A pocket rocket from M&S – effective, nourishing and wallet friendly.

- -

RoC Enydrial Repairing Lip Care €

This is a power lip balm and works when your lips are badly chapped, perhaps from medication, or just seriously dry. Seriously good and not badly priced at all.

- -

Nuxe Rêve de Miel Lip Balm €€

Free from artificial fragrances, preservatives and petroleum-based ingredients, this contains honey and shea butter to protect and nourish lips. Other gorgeous ingredients include grapefruit essential oil, so this smells good enough to eat.

- -

Cult Product: Cherry Chapstick €

Katy Perry shot this product into the stratosphere when she sang about kissing a girl and liking it. All of a sudden we were remembering the comforting presence of Chapstick and its wondrous ways. A real Product of Yore, this has been around for more than 100 years and is still going strong. It's available in numerous flavours and formulations – fruity, of course, and also minty, shimmery and SPF enriched. We're sure Russell approves.

Tip

Lip Treatment

Lip balm not cutting it and your lips still feel sore and dry? Try a lip treatment like Uriage Bariederm Lips overnight. Rich and super-moisturising, you'll notice a real difference in the morning.

Special Mention: Elizabeth Arden Eight Hour Cream €€€€

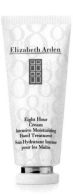

This little pot of wonder is a true cult product, and though it's not technically a lip balm, a lot of people use it as such. First magicked up by Elizabeth Arden in the 1930s as a salve for her racehorse's legs (no petroleum jelly for those babies), she realised just how good it was for humans too.

Containing ingredients including vitamin E and anti-inflammatory salicylic acid, it got the Eight Hour moniker due to a user who asserted that it fixed her son's scraped knee in – you guessed it – eight hours. One is sold every 2 minutes in the UK, and celebs like Cate Blanchett, Gisele Bundchen, Catherine Zeta-Jones, Claudia Schiffer, Victoria Beckham and Thandie Newton can't live without it, apparently.

Once you get past the smell, which a lot of people dislike, you'll find that this stuff works for chapped lips, grazes, small burns, unruly eyebrows, damaged cuticles and peeling skin. Make-up artists even employ it to give models a gorgeous sheen on skin.

The formula remains exactly the same now as it did the day Elizabeth Arden developed it and you can look out for the special editions with funky packaging – they bring these out all the time and they're great.

Beaut.ienomics:
Impulse Buying

Cosmetics could have been created by the Gods of Impulse Buying. They're small, beautiful – and expensive. Put a basket of lovely little things that no one needs beside the till and women will pick them up, examine them briefly – and add them to their shopping. It was chocolate at the supermarket till that did for us when we were children and it's the little bowls of sparkly stuff that do it for us now that we're adults.

We're in the mood, you see. We're in that shopping zone. And by the time we've reached the tills we're more likely to have thrown caution to the wind and abandoned ourselves to the giddy high of consumption. What is another tenner going to matter when you've already spent so much, after all? May as well be hung for sheep as for a lamb.

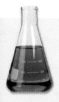

Read the Ingredients

Lip balm ingredients typically consist of things like petroleum jelly, beeswax, fats and vegetable oils. Each does different things – for example, wax in a lip balm acts like a cover, while vegetable oils help to soften lips.

Face Masks

There's nothing that says Pamper Time quite like a face mask. Slather some on, lie back and relax (cucumber slices over the eyes optional) and let it work – hard. A good mask should soothe, calm, deeply moisturise or purify. But most of all, we like masks because they give us a little time to ourselves to relax and wind down.

Recommendations

Shop Smart: Purity Organic Skincare Anti-ageing Serum and Mask €€

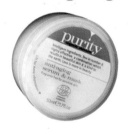

This little wonder is super-cheap and acts as both a hydrating mask and a shot of super-charged serum. Lash it onto dull skin for 10 minutes, wash off and reap the benefits. You'll have softer, smoother skin that'll feel nicely hydrated. This is great as a pick-me-up for skin that's tired and looking dull – and great for hangover skin too!

Shop Smart: Tesco Skin Wisdom Daily Care Detox Thermal Mask €

A good bargain bet for anyone with congested or oily skin, this contains clay, which draws out impurities and heats up on application for even more fancy shenanigans. It helps to scoop gunk out of pores, meaning they look a little tighter and it will leave skin looking fresh and clean.

Lush Oatifix €€

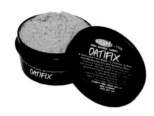

Like all of Lush's products, this is freshly made and packed full of natural ingredients. It smells like something you'd eat for breakfast (oats, bananas and almonds are all in the mix) and the name is obviously a pun on Oatibix. Oh, they're so wacky in Lush! This preparation is a thick paste that softens and nourishes and also contains illipe butter to reduce redness. A good all-rounder (but not recommended for those with very oily skin, as it can cause breakouts). Be warned: it must be kept in the fridge and goes off in about three weeks, so get ready to do a face mask every second night to use it all up.

Clarins Super Restorative Replenishing Comfort Mask €€€€€+

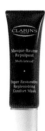

Developed for 50+ skin. Firming and hydrating, this mask is intensely moisturising and leaves skin silky smooth. Spread it over your face and neck and leave for 10 minutes. With ingredients like shea butter and mango, you can feel your skin calm and plump up. Clarins are masters of the whole silky smooth, perfect base for make-up style of skincare. If you like Dermalogica Multivitamin Power Recovery Masque, you'll like this too.

Soap & Glory No Clogs Allowed Deep Pore Detox Mask €€

Perfect for oily, congestion-prone skin, this comes with a little pink sponge for smooth application. It's a self-heating mask that warms up on your face, drawing out all those impurities and blamming spots and other nasty areas of congestion. It doubles up as an exfoliator too, so if you don't have the time or inclination for a mask, you can still get the benefits.

REN Glycolactic Skin Renewal Peel Mask €€€€€

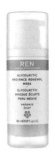

This gets absolutely rave reviews from Beaut.ie regulars, with many swearing that they cannot live without it. It's a particularly effective mix of fruit acids (glycolic, tartaric and citric) together with papain enzyme. Good for congested, blackhead-prone complexions, this orange gloop can also help to perk up a dull complexion. Because it's got quite a lot of active ingredients, we think sensitive skins might not get on too well with it.

Guaranteed Irish: Óg Ireland Peat Face Mask €€€€

With the consistency of a runny briquette, thankfully this doesn't smell of peat or muck and it works due to the fact that peat is packed with essential oils, fatty acids and lipids. These ingredients hydrate and help to re-establish the skin's natural pH balance. As it's detoxifying and anti-inflammatory, peat-based products are also reported to be beneficial for eczema, psoriasis and acne.

Body Shop Vitamin E Sink-In Moisture Mask €€

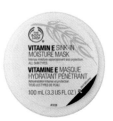

This is a bit of a best-kept backstage beauty secret with lots of make-up artists keeping one in their kits to pep up the skin of Fashion Week-ravaged models. Why? Cos it hydrates quickly, and as vitamin E is a great antioxidant, we think this is a good one to have on hand for those times when skin is dry, dull and stressed.

Cult Product: Dermalogica Multivitamin Power Recovery Masque €€€€

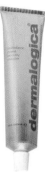

This is known on Beaut.ie as the 'orange burns victim mask' because that's exactly what you'll look like when you're wearing it – orange, dripping and disfigured. Not one to use in the first stages of a new relationship. However, it's probably the best-loved mask we've ever tried because it really packs a hydrating, juicy, delicious-smelling punch. Post-hangover when your skin feels dry and you woke up with your face stuck to the pillow thanks to last night's non-make-up-remover antics, it can give you an instant glow.

De-gunk First

You'll get the best out of any mask if you exfoliate first. It makes sense: if pores are clogged with dead skin, then the lovely nourishing, hydrating or purifying ingredients in your mask won't be able to properly penetrate and you won't get the full effect.

Spots

We hate them, but it's a fact that whether you're 14 or 40, spots have the capacity to make your life a living hell. We're well used to their kamikaze, lightning-strike ways and here's how we cope with them.

- All spot creams will dry out your skin – that's what they're designed to do – so don't use them for longer than you absolutely need to. Target them exactly on the spot itself – don't cover your whole chin with spot cream just to be sure.
- Don't poke, and if you really must pop a whitehead, make sure your hands are spotlessly clean and you don't dig about in the spot, causing bleeding. You really do run the risk of causing long-term damage to your face.

Recommendations

Shop Smart: Garnier Pure Active Spot-On Roll-On €

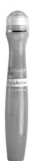

This roller ball yokey from Garnier has 2 per cent salicylic acid, which is a whizz for battling zits. It works – two days' application twice a day brings spots right down and almost completely fades redness.

Clearasil Ultra Rapid Action Treatment Cream €

Promising to reduce spot size and redness in just four hours, we were delighted to find that it actually does just that. Ingredients in the cream work to sink deep down into pores and shrink the nasty feckers. Definitely a handy one to have in the bathroom cabinet in case of emergencies.

Dermalogica Special Clearing Booster €€€€€

If your skin gets on well with Dermalogica products, chances are this is the spot treatment for you. It's strong: 5 per cent benzoyl peroxide plus other purifying ingredients will take no prisoners and blast spots into the stratosphere, where they belong.

The Doctor Brand Blemish Relief Kit €€€€€

This four-piece kit contains a cleanser, spot eliminator, pore-clearing gel and soothing lotion formulated with salicylic and glycolic acid to clear out blocked follicles. Make sure you lash on the moisturiser while using it – skin can become very dry while rebalancing – but this is definitely worth a try if you're at the end of your tether with spots.

Cult Product: Origins Spot Remover €€

Works fast and works well – salicylic acid and ingredients like oregano and clove battle with the spot and its nasty redness without drying out your skin too much. A good bet for those who find that Clearasil and the other teenage skin treatments are just too harsh.

Read the Ingredients

What should you look for in a zit zapper? Salicylic acid, sulphur and benzoyl peroxide are the wonder ingredients to look for.

Swap Siopa

This recession has seen the rise in popularity of clothes swapping parties and shops as people realised they had accumulated an enormous amount of clothes they didn't really need or want in more cash-rich times. And the same was true for beauty products, perfumes and cosmetics.

We set up Swap Siopa, an online beauty product exchange, on Beaut.ie for Irish women and it has turned out to be one of the most popular and well-used initiatives we've ever launched. With tens of thousands of visitors a month and new and lust-inducing swaps being posted on a daily basis, we were astonished at how busy it was right from the very beginning.

In reality, we shouldn't have been so surprised. Every woman has drawers and bathroom cabinets full of cosmetics and beauty products that were purchased in haste or received as gifts and then deemed unsuitable after a couple of uses. But because they've been opened and used, they can't be returned. Swap Siopa works so well because it ticks loads of boxes at once – it's free to join and no money ever changes hands, making it totally recession friendly. It's as green as they come – products that might have otherwise been added to landfill or left to moulder in a cupboard are sent to be used by someone who actively wants them.

Swap anything from skincare to bath and body products, make-up (but no used mascaras!) and that foundation that cost a fortune but the shade just didn't work on you.

So how does it work? You post your product on the forum or make someone else an offer if they've got something you'd like. When you're both happy, swap e-mail addresses so you can get contact details and post the stuff to one another. An Post carries your parcel off in one of its green vans and delivers it straight to your door. The whole thing is based on pure trust and in the years since Swap Siopa was established, we've had thousands of swaps completed.

In case you're not convinced yet, here's some feedback from our swappers.

Magpie says:

Well I was one of the first swappers on le Swap Siopa and overall it's fanfeckintastic. Any swaps I've had have been great:

- Products were as described
- Delivered ASAP
- Both got something they liked

Sure, what more could you ask for? Hurray for the Swap Siopa!

Amy says:

It's so addictive and you don't feel so guilty for the big splash-outs you made in the past! So glad to swap stuff that other people will appreciate and was just gathering dust in my make-up box!

Roxette says:

I bleedin' love the Swap Siopa! I've had countless swaps on it and have got to try stuff without spending more money, all the while getting rid of stuff that was gathering dust in my house. Haven't had one bad swap, which is a testament to all us lovely girls that use the site.

Also it makes me feel better that something I'm not using might be of use to someone else. I think everyone got a bit too extravagant and flippant with stuff during the Celtic Tiger and now that the recession is back people are actually appreciating more what they spend their money on.

Tbell says:

It's just great! I got rid of some things I really shouldn't have spent my money on and got some great stuff in return without a cent leaving the bank account! It puzzles my mum how I get all these packages arriving every week though ... I don't think she believes me that it's free!

salsera says:

I love Swap Siopa and have now got rid of all the eyeshadows that don't suit me, so I've nothing left to swap. I actually want a present that I don't like so I can get back in the game. How sad is that?

blacklashes says:

I forked out a wad of cash for Diorskin Nude foundation only to realise that I was an oompa loompa in natural light and needed the shade below ... thanks to Swap Siopa I was able to swap with another person who had bought the lighter shade and needed the one I had ... happy days! It's so difficult to know exactly how a product will work on you until you get it home and of course the minute you open it you can't take it back even though you've only swatched it! I check in with Swap Siopa every day.

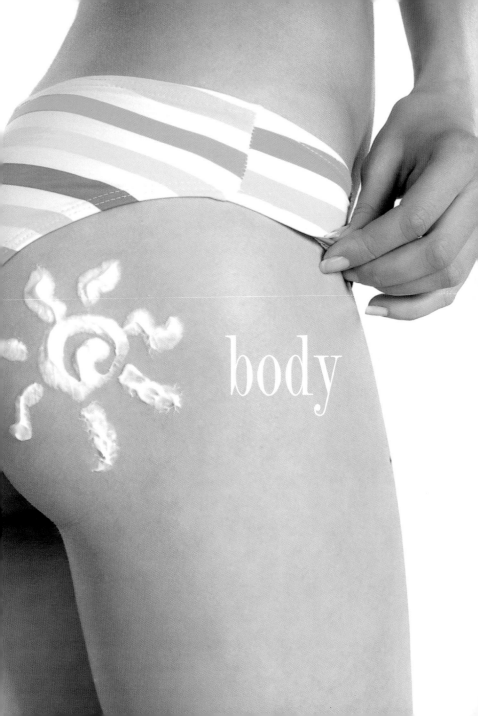

body

Hands

In order to stave off 'Madonna hands' for as long as possible (body of a teenager, hands of an octogenarian), slather on hand cream whenever you get a chance. Here's what we like.

Recommendations

Shop Smart: Sally Hansen 18 Hour Protective Hand Cream €€

It smells a bit medicinal, but this is lovely stuff. The consistency is rich, it's packed with nourishing goodies like shea butter and grapeseed oil and it goes a long way towards keeping hands smooth during the ravages of winter. Slathered on at night, it works really well to soften up *lamhas*.

Kiehl's Ultimate Strength Hand Salve €€

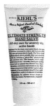

If you work outside, have your hands constantly in and out of water or have a manual job, you're going to need something really strong to treat your hands with. Lash some of this heavy-duty hand salve on. You'll feel the benefits of an application for hours and it will help to transform your roughened paws into actual hands again.

Love & Toast Hand Crème €€

Yummy flavours like mandarin and coconut and honey and adorable packaging make Love & Toast a winner with the young at heart. If you're a fan of the hand crème, you'll also love the pretty little tins of lip salve.

Neutrogena Norwegian Formula Hand Cream €

Hardworking, no prisoners taken, this is a bestselling hand cream classic that protects, softens and intensely moisturisers. No fuss, no fancy scents, this is Norwegian Formula, people – and they know all about cold-weather hands.

Body Shop Hemp Hand Protector €€

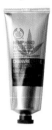

This Body Shop bestseller works really well. A high concentration of essential fatty acids helps to replenish moisture and leave hands soft.

Clinique Deep Comfort Hand and Cuticle Cream €€€

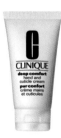

A hand and cuticle cream that's rich, soaks in quickly and doesn't leave hands feeling greasy. Fragrance free, it won't clash with your perfume.

No7 Protect & Perfect Hand Cream €€

A real workhorse cream, this protects your hands from the dreaded ageing and is a really good staple buy. The added SPF is a bonus too.

Soap & Glory Hand Food Hand Cream €

Smells delish (of course!), with extracts of fennel and lotus flower. Light and non-greasy, it's a perfect present. Pick this up in three for two sales and it will last for ages.

Cult Product: Clarins Hand and Nail Treatment Cream €€

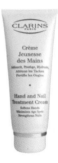

This stuff is the business. It's been around for yonks and is a product that women absolutely fall in love with and repurchase time and time again. Loads of nourishing and hydrating goodies are in here, like sesame oil extracts, shea butter, Japanese mulberry extract and myrrh extract to strengthen nails. Not the cheapest, of course, but widely regarded to be one of the best – try some for yourself.

Marcel Marceau

For extra hydration and hardworkingness, slather on cream before bed and then pop some cotton gloves on (you'll find these at Boots or the Body Shop) over the top. Ignore the derisive sniggering of your flatmates or other half and get your zeds, content that in the morning you'll have soft, smooth paws and they'll have hands that resemble bark, with loads of hangnails to boot.

Feet

Generally the yuckiest parts of most people's bodies, feet have a terrible old life. Stuffed into too-tight shoes and smelly runners, who can be surprised they look horrible most of them time? Give them some love by using a proper foot moisturiser and getting rid of the yellow bits (ugh).

Recommendations

Aveda Foot Relief €€€

Good old Foot Relief has been around for yonks and still manages to outrun most of its competition. Botanical oils moisturise, fruit acids exfoliate gently to nibble off dead skin and essential oils of lavender, rosemary and peppermint refresh and soothe tired feet.

Flexitol Heel Balm €

Cheap and brilliant. Flexitol is chocca with urea, the active ingredient that softens skin. With 7 per cent urea it's one of the strongest over-the-counter topical creams you can buy. Goodbye, cheese rind hooves!

Ped Egg €€

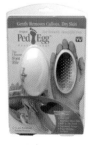

Who would have thought that something so cheap and naff looking from JML could be so downright brilliant? The Ped Egg took the world by storm as everyone enjoyably grated all the old horrible yellow cheesy skin off their trotters. The shocking evidence of these gratings remain trapped in the egg until it's emptied, leaving feet softly shaven.

Use Your Foot Cream on Your Elbows

We were horrified to read that elbows are one of the big barometers of ageing. Possibly one of the most neglected parts of the body, elbows can make you look ancient from behind. One of the best tips we've gotten is to use your foot cream on your elbows. Cheap and very effective, that tough old skin will be sorted out in a trice.

Read the Ingredients

● Shea Butter

This is the ingredient that makes any cosmetic that contains it so luxurious and moisturising. It's a natural ingredient and comes from the karite tree. Natural and richly hydrating, it's a winner.

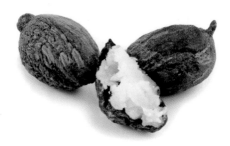

Body Wash

If there's one thing we get through in bucketloads – or at least I hope we do – it's shower gel, wash or soap.

To be honest, this is one area where own brand really comes into its own. You can scrimp with abandon on three for twos and buy one get one free and indulge in all the lovely scents by buying at the right time.

Recommendations

Shop Smart: Tesco Wake Up €

Such a blatant copy of the Original Source shower gels, we don't know how they're getting away with it – but they are. Half the price of the zingy original, this is a fantastic shower gel – orange and ginger and lemon and mint are unisex scents that will revive anyone.

Spoil Me Naked Coco de Mer Bath Foam €

With a bit of an oooh-er message on the label about erotic potential, sharing a naked bath and steamy nights, we instantly hurried to try out this bath foam. Sadly, none of this happened, but we did like this bubble bath very much and its coconut fragrance is well worth filling the tub for – even if you are *sniffle* on your own.

Boots Botanics Luxurious Bath Elixir €

Mmmm, if you love the smell of Botanics products (and we do), you're on to a winner with this bath foam. With Iceland moss, this promises to soothe and relax away stress and strain and ease tired muscles. For only a few quid it certainly does that and smells delicious to boot.

Tisserand Energy Revive Bath Oil €€

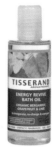

Bergamot, grapefruit and lime organic oils combine to provide a zesty blend that's perfect for a reviving bath.

A great wake-up – or we've found it's brilliant when you've come home from work tired and need to rev back up for a night out to kick start the engines.

Roger & Gallet Rose Moisturizing Fragrant Shower Cream €€

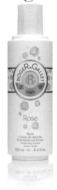

Only mad into their garden analogies they are in R&G. They reckon this shower cream will lead you to the garden of the Sultan's palace in India and wrap you in softness like a Bengalese sari. Well, we don't know about that – but we do know that this shower cream is deliciously and headily scented and is rich and creamy in texture – it's a sumptuous treat.

Vichy Essentielles Shower Gel €

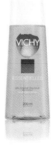

Part of Vichy's affordable Essentielles line, this shower gel is nicely rose scented and is kind to dry and sensitive skin types. Hypoallergenic and paraben free, it's a real daily essential. Geddit?

Beaut.ienomics:
Own Brand Copycat

M&S do a great line in Body Shop 'homages' and they're usually nice and packaged well. Marks & Spencer actually do a great line in copying everything. A quick glance over their shelves reveals scarily similar packaging to quite a few well-known brands, including L'Oréal Paris, Neutrogena, Clarins and of course the Body Shop. It's a shame, because when they do try to be original, they usually do it well – the Tess Daly range is a case in point. But they still have the dubious honour of being the best place to buy talc sets and royal jelly-themed bath and body products. So that's good anyway.

Smellies Make Great Gifts, But Use with Caution

'Smelly' is a term for any bath or shower product that you give as a present. As in 'I'm just popping in to the Body Shop to pick up some smellies to add to my sister's present', or 'Oh, I hope someone gives me smellies for Christmas, I'm right out of bath bombs.'

Be careful with smelly gifting, however – they can signify thoughtlessness on a big scale if not chosen with, er, thought. Man smellies have virtually replaced socks as a staple gift for all those tiresome occasions that blokes must be given presents. And let's face it: men are very difficult to buy for. Pity the man who gets four identical Lynx box sets at Christmas though. Spray more, get more, eh?

Cult Product: Lush Bath Bombs €

We have a bit of a love–hate relationship with Lush. We do like their natural ethos and their wackily named products, but we have a slight problem with the smell sometimes. Lush don't do subtle. They do 'hit you over the head and pound you into submission' with the whiff of some of their offerings. Plus their 'freshly made' cosmetics have a desperate tendency to go off before you get a chance to finish them. That aside, we do love some of their bath and body bits.

Lush Bath Bombs are copied so much that they're most definitely a cult product, and some of their new shower gels aren't half bad either (stand up Flying Fox Shower Gel). If you like strong scents, you're on to a winner with Lush.

Recommendations

Shop Smart: Lidl Suhada Nature €

Not a lot of people know this, but Lidl has a really good natural bath and body range – Suhada Nature. They aren't tested on animals, are free from artificial perfume, colours and chemicals and adhere to strict organic guidelines. Certified by BDIH, the German equivalent of the UK's Soil Association, you're guaranteed products that are nasty free and kind to the earth. And as befits Lidl's ethos, they're super-cheap too. Think under a fiver for a lot of the range and you won't be far wrong.

Problem is that a lot of products are released as limited editions and in store for a certain time only – until they sell out, basically, so when you see something you like, snap up a few of them.

Based on price, this range knocks the socks off most natural offerings. If we're honest, we think it's worth swapping your Dr Hauschka and Lavera for Suhada Nature. Possibly the only difference you'll notice is in your purse. We likey.

Kneipp Herbal Body Wash Rosemary €€

Kneipp is a German organic brand that is certified to the teeth and a great choice if you like pure and natural products with more than a touch of ethical about them.

Body Shop Sweet Lemon Shower Gel €

It smells delish and not too sweet and is a really nice way to wake up in the morning, especially if your morning routine is anything like ours: arise from bed in zombie fashion, mumbling and grumbling, feeling our way by touch to the bathroom because we can't yet bear to open our eyes. Too much information? But you get the drift – this is great.

Organic Surge €

Yummy scrummy: this range comes in all manner of delicious smells and is almost organic (despite the name, it's not actually certified). But you can rest assured that over 95 per cent of the ingredients are organic. There are loads of 'flavours', but the Tropical Bergamot is a winner and the Citrus Mint might just be the thing for the man in your life.

· ·

Read the Ingredients

● Mint

Mint is often used in bath and shower products and enthusiastically proclaims itself as a fabulous energising ingredient. Be careful of any mint washes near your, er, nethers though. You may get more of a zing than you'd expected. Or as one gentleman confided in me when discussing one particularly spearminty offering, 'This stuff would freeze the mickey off you.' Right so!

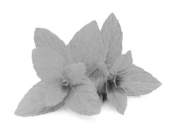

Body Creams and Scrubs

2010 was the year when lots of body products were launched, each with more startling claims than the other. The first one promised to penetrate three layers deep into the skin (Vaseline Sheer Infusion, how are ya). Grand so, we thought, that sounds fine. But as successive products were launched to rival this we were worried that we might actually be moisturising our, er, bones.

It was also the year of falling in love with dry oils — read on and we'll tell you more.

Recommendations

Shop Smart: Vaseline Sheer Infusion €

This range of body lotions works on a triple threat basis — they work their way down through three layers of skin and the formula holds four times more moisture than a normal glycerin-based lotion. Even better, it soaks in really quickly, so no wuthering tights and within five minutes you can put your stockings on.

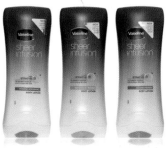

Shop Smart: Nivea Body Firming Body Lotion Q10 Plus €

Now, don't expect this to smell as pretty as your fancy pants scented body lotions: just expect this to be a damn good workhorse. Spreads on the skin well, sinks in like a dream and applied after a daily shower it really does seem to firm up skin. Cheap as anything and really good. Give this a go instead of shelling out for expensive cellulite creams – there's no proof yet that any of them actually work, but you can hedge your bets with this boyo.

Neutrogena Deep Moisture Body Lotion and Deep Moisture Comfort Balm €

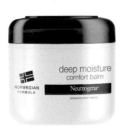

So you thought Vaseline Sheer Infusion was doing well? Neutrogena say this body moisturiser penetrates 10 layers down into the stratum corneum – the top layer of the skin. We were a bit worried in case the cream could sink down as far as bone, but we were just being silly apparently. These are lightweight, hardworking skin creams that provide a decent barrier and include lots of emollients and humectants to give skin hydration.

Roger & Gallet Huile Sublime Bois D'Orange €€€

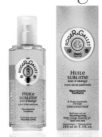

A beautiful dry oil from this French brand. The scent is absolutely astounding – fresh, citrusy and with more mellow orange than we would have thought possible. Mandarin orange, bergamot, verbena and orange blossom are all blended into a fragrance that is not overpowering, just warm and summery and delicious.

Garnier Intensive 7 Days Body Lotion €

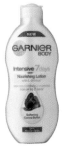

With five delish 'flavours' to choose from there really is one for everyone in the audience. Every type of skin is catered for – from sensitive down to as dry and crackly as an overdone rasher. And the technology promises us that we'll feel the benefits for a whole seven days after application. This might be going a bit too far: suffice it to say that this range rocks and is at a great price point. Watch out for it on special offer too. Garnier often discount their products, so you'll get it even cheaper.

Kiehl's Crème de Corps €€€€

Kiehl's sparked a frenzy when they finally set up shop on our shores. Every stylish gal has a bottle of Crème de Corps on her bathroom shelf – gorgeous stuff, it's creamy and highly moisturising. And we also like the fact that Kiehl's made it a priority to keep their Irish prices as close to their US ones as possible.

Soap & Glory The Righteous Butter Body Lotion €€

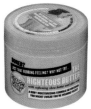

If you love a rich, thick and sweet-smelling cream, then you'll love this. Not only is the retro packaging adorable, the contents find high favour with our readers who rate this body butter as their all-time great.

E45 Endless Moisture Radiance €€

This is a new and improved version of the beloved E45 body mosituriser with all the long-lasting, hypoallergenic hydration of the original in the same lightweight, non-greasy formula. But this has been fabulised with subtle sparkly bits. The sparkly bits are very understated though, so no worrying about accidentally resembling a disco ball – you'll just glow prettily.

Clarins Extra-Firming Body Cream €€€€€+

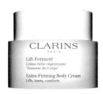

So thick it's almost like a body butter in texture, so velvety smooth you can almost feel it sinking in and so good for skin you'll notice an immediate effect. It's made with lemon thyme and other delicious ingredients to help skin that's become saggy and baggy due to pregnancy, weight changes or just downright ageing. Or all of them. Yummy.

Cult Buy: Nuxe Huile Prodigieuse €€

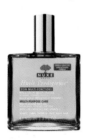

Notice the dry oil theme going on here? We've fallen truly, madly, deeply in love with these dry guys. This is one of our all-time winter skin savers. Spray on before bed, under moisturiser and into hands and nails and use to clear up annoying dry patches of skin. It also works mixed with foundation to make it more moisturising and into hair to smooth down frizzy bits— there is literally no end to its wonders.

Trend: Temporary Tattoos

If you thought these were naff, think again. Although our memories of temporary tattoos are blighted by childhood memories of the ones free with chewing gum, we have been reconsidering their appeal. As soon as Chanel released their 'temporary skin art' Les Trompe-L'Oeil, tattoos became less Britney Spears and more Juliet Binoche. Strings of pearls, jewelled birds with Chanel logos in their beaks and sprays of flowers all abounded, but they were a bit expensive for everyone's taste.

Cheaper copies soon became available as other brands jumped on the bandwagon, meaning everyone could have a go. So let's have a bit of fun – if the normally stuffy Chanel can, surely we can too?

Read the Ingredients

The Paraben Controversy

If there was ever a case of scaremongering, this is it. There's a lot of misinformation about the benefits of natural cosmetics over synthetically formulated ones. We're told that chemicals are evil and natural is the only way to go, even though most of the chemicals used in regulated cosmetics are 100 per cent safe. Parabens are probably the most famous example of this. Used as preservatives in cosmetics, parabens are included in cream and liquid formulations to ensure that any nasties like MRSA don't flourish in what would otherwise be a very nice moist and welcoming environment. The chemical parabens which are used in beauty products are synthesised versions of those found in nature – blueberries contain a lot of them, for example, and that's why they last so long.

Where It All Came From

In 2004 a report suggested that parabens used in antiperspirants might be responsible for some cases of breast cancer. But it was a big might: the research was flawed and the conclusions drawn didn't stand up. It was enough to kick start the whole paraben controversy though, which ignited like a Bord na Móna fire log and now burns so fiercely not even a hunky fireman could put it out.

While cosmetic scientists would like a proper study to be undertaken once and for all to find out if parabens are harmful or not, this hasn't yet happened. So while there's no actual proof that they're harmful, equally what's true is that there's no hard and fast proof they're completely safe and that they don't cause cancer.

If you want to avoid them you'll find increasing numbers of products labelled paraben free on the shelves, and that's not just restricted to green cosmetics any more. Brands like Lancôme and Vichy are increasingly releasing new launches that don't include them and brands like Jergens are creating new forms of safe preservatives too. We're not too bothered about parabens ourselves, but we do applaud companies for looking into new forms of preservatives – after all, choice is good, eh?

Stretch Marks

Stretch marks can occur at any time — with puberty, weight gain, certain medicine and especially pregnancy. Most women have them – and if you don't you're a lucky bunny.

The jury is out on whether they're actually just down to genetics and therefore if topical treatments (creams to you and me) will actually do any good, but to be honest, slathering yourself in product can't actually do any harm and may make you feel a lot better about the nasty things

The problem is that any product can claim to reduce and improve the look of stretch marks — and very few of them actually do it. Despite what any label may claim, there is really only one time to tackle them: when they're still red. Once they fade to silver there is precious little that can be done without recourse to heavier-duty treatments. And as always, prevention is better than cure. If you're really desperate, you can think about having Fraxel. A medical laser, Fraxel is effective but it's painful, expensive and you'll probably need to endure a course of treatment.

Trilogy Rosehip Oil €€

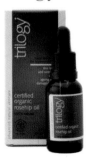

The number one stretch mark preventer used by pregnant Beaut.ie readers. Certified organic, this oil has actually been clinically proven to prevent stretch marks and aid in their healing. Independent clinical trials found that scars were reduced by 41 per cent and stretch marks were reduced by 43 per cent. Organic and packed with natural ingredients, it comes in a 45ml bottle, ideal for body.

Palmers Cocoa Butter Scar Serum €€

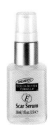

This is a highly concentrated version of cocoa butter oil together with other oils. Not just for stretch marks, this will work to tackle any type of scarring – try using it on caesarean scars too.

StriVectin €€€€€+

It's not often the same product is as good for the arse as it is for the face: this is the exception. See p. 14 in the Anti-ageing section for more on this.

Cult Product: Palmers Cocoa Butter Skin Therapy Oil €€

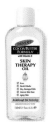

You'll smell like a Snickers – but a delicious yummy mummy one. A variation on the well-known cream is Palmers Cocoa Butter Skin Therapy Oil: a light and intensely moisturising oil that leaves skin silky smooth and glowing. It also comes in a non-scented version – handy to know if you feel nauseous during pregnancy.

Scrubs

Although cynics will tell you that all body scrubs are basically just grit in some kind of cream or oil, we disagree. All scrubs are not created equal – and the following are rated again and again for the pure pleasure of their use, for their scent and their effectiveness. With the exception of the Clinique product, all are low or mid-price so won't cost the earth and will help to firm and smooth skin.

Soap & Glory The Scrub of Your Life €

Johnson's Bodycare Gentle Exfoliating Body Wash €

Lush Buffy the Backside Slayer €€

Body Shop Olive Oil Scrub €€

Sanctuary Hot Sugar Scrub €€

Cult Product: Clinique Sparkle Skin €€€€

Beaut.ienomics:
Oh Baby Baby

Babies: you are responsible for being much more than being cute and adorable. You might not realise it as you gurgle sweetly away in your cot, but you are directly to blame for getting your mother hooked on natural skincare and cosmetics.

Women want to do the absolute best for the new little life growing inside of them, so as soon as they know that they're pregnant, most of them start on a health regime the likes of which they've never been inspired to do before. Out goes anything with the slightest whiff of chemicals in case it will cause harm.

This is a natural reaction and the cosmetic industry preys on this fear. It is used as the perfect time to make you pregnant ladies all hyper-worried about the effects of chemicals, preservatives and additives in cosmetics. This is a great opportunity to push you over to the more expensive side of natural and organic cosmetics – which, naturally, are very profitable. So, during pregnancy, women are seduced into believing that organic is the only way to go and many of them stick with this expensive belief for a long time.

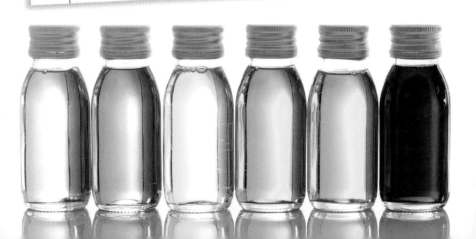

Tan

We've got a *grá* for tan in Ireland, that's for sure. We don't get very much sun stuck out on a rainy little island on the edge of Europe, and as we all know, summer can consist of one good week. This is why we need to fake it up if we are to get any colour at all. Irish women are so fond of fake tan that we use 60 per cent more of it than our nearest neighbours, the UK.

But herein lies the rub. We're very pale and most tan is not formulated to suit our skin tone. Orange tans and foundation tidemarks are something for which we're known abroad – the shame.

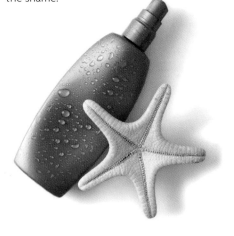

 ## Go Gradual

As a general rule, gradual tan is a winner for Irish and Polish skin. Because the colour is buildable you can make sure that you don't apply more than you need. Go as brown as you would naturally – and no more. You hear us now?

Beaut.ienomics:
Shop Around

Johnson & Johnson got in there first with supermarket gradual tan. When their Holiday Skin burst onto the market, we all went crazy for it. (Never mind that it stank and went a worrying colour after a couple of applications.) They've improved the formulation now though: it smells fresher and wears off better.

But like any good idea, it was copied, and copied with a vigour and enthusiasm that can only mean one thing: there's money to be made in them thar fake tanned hills. Serious money is to be made using a process that essentially is as simple as lobbing some colour activator into a cheap body lotion.

Because there are so many players in the market, there are significant savings to be had. Fake tan is a beauty shelf staple and that means that tan is as heavily discounted as shampoo or deodorant. You should never pay full price for your shot of bronze – three for twos and buy one get one free are popular options here.

Fake tan is actually a desperate product. It's proven impossible to make it smell nice, it's a nightmare to apply and you practically need a degree in tanning to make it look natural. And even if you reckon you've done enough home applications to have gained that degree, it only takes one bad application to land you back in the streak central detention pen.

Word is that sales of tan have dropped and we predict that this craze has hit its peak, so feel free to embrace your inner Dita Von Teese.

Salon tanning has drastically come down in price as salons offer spray tanning much more cheaply – and so they should, it's a very low-cost treatment for them. Look out for offers that include waxing or eyebrow shaping thrown in with the colour.

Recommendations

Shop Smart: Dove Summer Glow Gradual Fake Tan €

This supermarket gradual tan is very popular on Beaut.ie. It's easy to apply, easy to build and it's hard to go wrong with a gradual tan, so it's good for novices. It takes the corned beef look off the palest of skin and is reasonably priced.

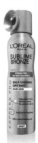

Shop Smart: L'Oréal Sublime €€

Probably the best of the mass market tans, this has lots of variations, making it a sure bet that you'll find a formulation to suit you. Amy Huberman is reputed to have worn this on her wedding day – we don't know if that's true or not, but that says a lot for its reputation.

Shop Smart: St Moritz for Penneys €

Unbelievably, a tan costing less than €3 is making the grade here. St Moritz (wonder where they got that name, eh?) is a mousse-based tan that you can build to give a depth of colour and it gets much love on Beaut.ie.

Guaranteed Irish: Tan Organic €€€€

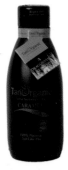

An Irish *Dragons' Den* success story, this home-grown tan is great if you want a dark colour. It's a liquid, which can be a bit of a pain to apply, as it's messy and can splash on places that don't need to be tanned – like your duvet or your new white towels. The professional salon spray tan version is a far better option and gives even, natural-looking colour.

Other Irish tans are He-Shi, Wow Brown and Rockstar Tan. If you feel like being patriotic with your bit of bronze, give one of these a whirl.

Clarins Instant Smooth Self Tanning €€€

This really is a pot of tanning magic. Apply it over the top of your other face products – moisturiser/SPF and the like – and watch as it gives you a bronze glow that develops and builds every day you use it. It's a face tan that feels like a primer and works like one to smooth out lines and instantly fabulise you.

Xen-Tan Deep Bronze Luxe €€€

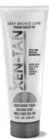

If you're paler than pale and still want to try your hand at a deep tan, this gets good feedback. It has a nice olive tone (as opposed to the violent orange of many of its competitors), so it looks quite natural. Apply one coat for a medium tan and two for deep.

St Tropez Rapide Face €€€

The problem with using a body tan on your phizog is the clogged pores you'll accumulate as a result – big durty brown ones. That's why you need to be careful and just use a tan formulated especially for the face. St Tropez Rapide Face is one of the best.

Tess Daly Body Sheen €€

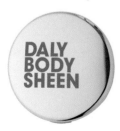

A little sweep of shimmer across the collarbones, décolletage or legs can look absolutely gorgeous. Another Tess Daly product works well here: Daly Body Sheen is a sheer highlighter for use on the body. You won't get coverage with this one, but you will get a shimmering, dewy glow.

Rimmel Sun Shimmer €

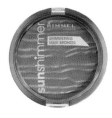

If you prefer to brush on your bronze, there are two great powder compacts to choose from in the Sun Shimmer range. The big Maxi Bronzer is a winner and is loaded with golden shimmer. If you'd like a matte bronzer and a more intense colour, go for the original Sun Shimmer compact.

Nuxe Huile Prodigieuse Shimmer Dry Oil €€€€

A version of the classic Nuxe Huile Prodigieuse Dry Oil (see p. 84) containing gorgeous golden particles, this is easy to apply and will enhance any tan, either real or from a bottle.

Bobbi Brown Shimmer Brick €€€

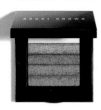

Great if you want a bit of shimmer and want to enhance those oh-so-sexy collarbones and shoulders – brush on some body shimmer and give yourself an instant glow. Take a look at the Blusher, Bronzer and Highlighter section on pp. 159–64 for more recommendations.

Cult Product: Sally Hansen Airbrush Legs €€

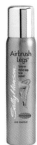

Legs are probably the most difficult part of the body to fake tan successfully. Streaky calves, muddy knees and dirty protest shins are commonly reported. Thankfully, this product never fails to impress. Like stockings for legs, it's easy to apply, gives impressive results and doesn't streak or wash off in the rain.

Read the Ingredients

Dihydroxyacetone (DHA)

Every bottle of fake tan that develops on the skin has one ingredient in common – they all contain dihydroxyacetone (DHA) as the active component. DHA is a sugar that reacts in a chemical process when applied to the skin. This is what causes the change in colour and it's also what causes the horrid digestive biscuit smell. It's a colourless ingredient in itself, but as it interacts with these cells, a colour change occurs that is closer to orange than brown, which is why it's so difficult to get a fake tan that turns a nice natural bronze.

We don't believe brands that claim to have a smell-free formulation, because if what they're offering is a tan that develops, then they're using DHA to do it and as we noted above, it smells to high heaven.

Beaut.ienomics:
Pick Skin-finishing Products

Irish women are changing the way they use fake tan. The trend is much more towards a lighter, more natural finish that will wash off at the end of the evening.

The brands that have already cottoned on to this are making a killing. Rimmel's Sun Shimmer Maxi Instant Tan is selling like hotcakes: cheap and plentiful (it comes in a 250ml pump), it's the ideal solution for someone who wants colour quickly.

MAC Face and Body Foundation and Make Up For Ever Face & Body have been around for millions of years and are both fantastic skin-finishing staples. Gosh Instant Tan Gel is available in two shades, light and medium, and is a lightweight bronze gel that blends really well, leaving just a hint of colour. St Tropez Wash Off Instant Glow Body lotion is also a decent wash-off tint.

Pretty much the entire Tess Daly line for Marks & Spencer was created with skin finishing in mind. Daly Light is for use on the face, but it will also work on arms and chest. You could try mixing it with a bit of MAC Face and Body to give it more coverage and shimmer.

Sun Protection

With an alarmingly high rate of skin cancer and a skin type that goes from zero to sunburned in 60 seconds (thank you, David Murray), we Irish badly need to use suncreams. So you'd think it would be safe to assume that this is one area immune to the dip in consumption we're seeing in some other categories. Not so. We're going on fewer holidays and it seems that because of this, we have less use for those tubes of suncream.

We still need protection though, even if staycations are what we're doing now. An Irish summer's day is enough to turn most of us into a boiled lobster if not properly protected and an SPF of at least 15 is recommended to stave off sun ageing.

Beaut.ienomics: Choose Own Brand Sunscreen

This is one area where you can really save money – cut-price suncare can be every bit as good in protection terms as expensive versions. Just make sure it carries certification marks to ensure quality. Your Aldi sunscreen will keep you as well protected as a Sisley product – and cost a hell of a lot less.

Recommendations

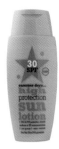

Shop Smart: Penneys SPF 30 Sun Lotion €

This sinks in well, has broad-spectrum protection at a high SPF level and it's at such a low price that you really don't have any excuse not to be slapping on the sunscreen.

Garnier Ambre Solaire Golden Protect Oil SPF 30 €€€

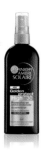

Oil on the skin is really flattering, particularly if the oil is slightly tinted – it instantly makes you look summery and glowy. This oil has been knocking around for decades, but due to sciencey difficulties it never had a high sun protection factor included until recently. Golden Protect Oil is enriched with shea butter for maximum moisturisation and has a high SPF factor (available up to SPF 30).

Boots Soltan Invisible Dry-Touch Transparent Suncare Spray €€

The brilliant nozzle means that this bottle even sprays upside down, meaning that you can spray all those hard-to-reach areas (er, let's not consider this one too much) and your lightning-fast children from any angle. It's transparent (no greasy white lotion to rub in) and water resistant – spray it on, put on your sundress and you're good to go.

RoC Minesol Sun Protection Fluid Cream SPF 50 €€

RoC is a brand famous for keeping things looking as young as possible, and their suncreams are no different. They're formulated to minimise allergies and contain ingredients to help stimulate the natural skin defence processes to help maintain 'cell integrity'. A cell with integrity seems like a cell that's been brought up properly and we like the sound of that.

Clarins UV Plus HP Multi-Protection Day Screen SPF 40 €€€€

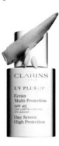

If you don't like putting chemicals on your face, this 100 per cent mineral sunscreen will suit you down to the ground. Apply it over the top of your regular moisturiser and let the minerals (like titanium dioxide and aluminium) physically block out the sun's rays. There's a bit of antioxidant action going on too, so it will also help to fight the effects of pollution.

Shiseido Urban Environment UV Protection Cream €€€€

More pricey than the others we're rating, but if you're looking for a sunscreen to wear on a daily basis (rather than on trips to the beach, for instance), this will suit you down to the ground. If you like Clinique City Block, you're going to love this — it has a much nicer texture and feel, is comfortable to wear on a daily basis and won't block your pores.

Cult Product: La Roche-Posay Anthelios XL SPF50+ €€€

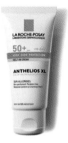

Absolutely the best sunscreen with a factor of 50+ for use on the face. It won't react with even the most sensitive of skin and works well as a base under make-up. Get the tinted version if you want to go make-up free.

Beaut.ienomics:
The Lure of Store Layouts

We all know why the milk and bread are at the back of the supermarket – the devilish people who plan store layout do it to make us walk the whole way through and pick up other items on the way.

Well, just like the supermarkets, the cosmetics halls and chemists are structured in similar ways. It's the Ikea model of store layout – make you trudge through the whole store before you can actually get to what you want, planting the seeds for delicious wanting and needing along the way.

Running to Boots for a packet of Paracetamol? Let's take the Liffey Valley store as an example. A sensory overload awaits you, tempting you in every way possible with colours, expensive products, bargains galore and new, as yet untried products. You'll have to pass by:

- The banners proclaiming special offers. (Oh look! 500 extra points on all No7 purchases!)
- The premium beauty counters. (Oh look! It's Clinique Bonus Time!)
- The cosmetics, with their end of bay point of sale (Oh look! That new Maybelline mascara!) and skincare deals (Oh look! My Olay Regenerist at half price!).
- The staple buys. (Oh look! Three for two on the Sure deodorant I use!)
- The hair care. (Oh look! Buy one get one free on my shampoo!)

At last, you're in the boring back of the shop with the prescriptions and the painkillers and the nappies and cotton wool. It's noticeably quieter and less frantic here, so use this as an opportunity to take a breather, because you have to run the assault course all over again as you make your way back up to the tills at the front of the store.

I hope you grabbed a basket on your way in, because you'll need it as you stagger back up through the store, basket groaning under the weight of all the things you didn't even know you needed. But you've just saved so much, haven't you? Well, haven't you?

Is it any wonder that Boots Liffey Valley is their highest-grossing store in all of the entire UK and Ireland?

Rip-off Ireland

Rip-off Ireland is alive and well and living in your bathroom cabinet

When Gordon Gekko said 'greed is good', he might as well have been talking about the behaviour of the beauty industry in Ireland rather than stockbrokers on Wall Street.

Cosmetic pricing in Ireland is totally off the scale. We pay more in Ireland. Brands rack up their profit margin and hide it when challenged by muttering about the exchange rate and the cost of doing business in Ireland.

Rubbish. Absolute rubbish.

We need parity of pricing, or as close to it as possible. We're in a horrible recession and we cannot afford to pay these jacked-up mark-ups any longer. When our prices are compared with those of the UK, the US and other European countries, the differences are astounding. There's absolutely no reason for it – apart from greed and the fact that they can get away with it.

When we started to write about beauty pricing seriously, there was already mass consumer dissatisfaction with grocery and clothing prices. They received plenty of media attention, and as a result of intense consumer pressure prices are slowly beginning to fall. Cosmetic prices never really got this attention and as a result are as high as ever.

Beaut.ie never shuts up about the price differential between Ireland and other markets. We have been shouting about it from the rooftops for years. We've done price comparisons, we've identified the brands that are the worst offenders (for the record, it's not always the high-end brands, it's mostly the big mass market brands) and we've consistently asked brands directly why they are shoving such a big mark-up on products sold in Ireland.

Let's do something about it. Go online and sign our petition to lower cosmetic prices in Ireland. Tell us how you feel about it on the Beaut.ie forums.

Notes

Notes

Notes

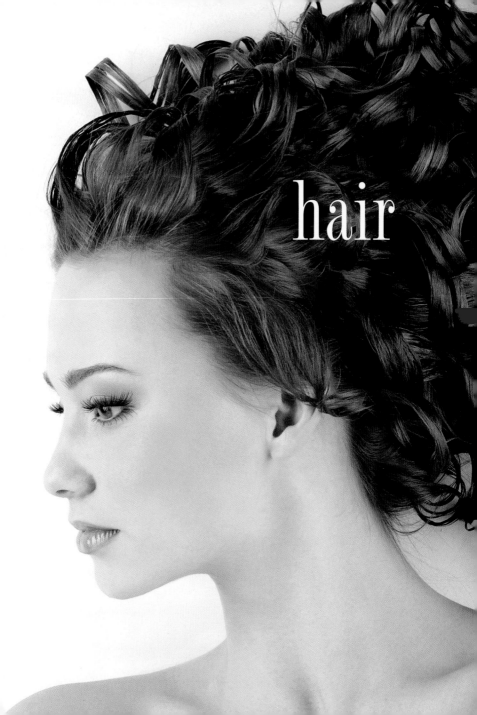

hair

Hair Care Essentials

Women have simple needs. We need food, shelter and hair care.

The hair care market in Ireland is worth about €140 million, but it's one of the beauty areas that is being hard hit by the recession. It's really easy to save money on hair care, you see. Budget brands have improved and we've traded down from salon treatments and are now doing much more at home. Happily, DIY colour has become much easier to use and less heavy on the chemicals. As a result, we're colouring at home far more these days.

The hair care industry is fighting back, though — we've seen the introduction of expensive treatments like the permanent blow dry, a craze for hair oils and new styling and treatment products. Reductions in salon prices and special offers have become commonplace and have ensured that women have kept going to the hairdresser. Not as much as they would have done, sure, but let's face it: there's nothing better than getting your hair done, is there? Especially if the price is lower.

When it comes down to it, women love their hair so much, they will do literally anything to keep it looking good. The fat is being drastically trimmed from this sector and only the strong will survive. We need to demand value.

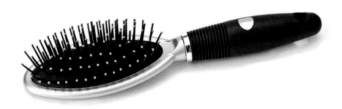

Beaut.ienomics:
Staple Buys

Shampoo is one of the products that is regarded as a staple buy. We can (in theory) cut down on other things that we don't actually need, like make-up, but we need to be clean. Therefore, shampoo is a must-have, like deodorant and shower gel, and purchased by men and women alike. These are part of the social requirements of modern life – we need to be hygienic. So recognised are these needs that cosmetic companies fight tooth and nail to get a foothold in this sector and value turnover and quantity.

So what does this mean for you, the consumer? Value. Bargains, and lots of them. Buy one get one free, three for two, 50 per cent extra free, buy one thing get this free, introductory offers – they're all here.

Which is glorious for the consumer. If you're a fan of mass market shampoos (anything from John Frieda and Pantene to Head and Shoulders and VO5), then there is no need for you to ever pay full price for your shampoo and conditioner again. Either stockpile when offer time comes around or try out new brands when you see them on offer.

Recommendations

Shop Smart: L'Oréal Elvive Damage Rescue Intensive Conditioner €

With all sorts of fancy science and technology (including something excitingly called hair cement), this promised much and delivered much. Surprisingly good for such a cost-effective product, if you've used and abused your poor *gruaig* with heat, over-styling and colour, then give it a break with a good dollop of this deep conditioner.

Pantene Pro-V Aqua Light €

If you've got fine hair that often feels weighed down and slightly sticky after regular shampoo, this range is ideal because of its Clean Rinse formula — there's no residue left behind afterwards to limpen locks.

Plenty of us avoided Pantene in the past because it gave shiny, glossy hair initially but became dull with product build-up. This range doesn't do this because they've tinkered around with the formula, reducing the amount of heavy silicones and making it much more suitable for fine hair.

L'Oréal Paris Elvive Full Restore 5 €

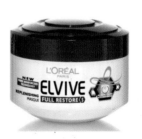

Yes, this is the one that Cheryl Cole advertises so prettily, and while you may not have the hair extensions to get her look, this range really does deliver. The shampoo, conditioner and masque in the Full Restore 5 line are chock full of pro-keratin to reinforce hair and leave it better able to resist daily wear and tear and ceramides to smooth the surface of the hair and add softness and shine. Really good stuff and now a staple on our bathroom shelves.

Head & Shoulders Hydrating Smooth & Silky €

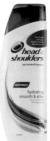

No one was more surprised than we were to discover that we actually really like this shampoo and conditioner. After years of scoffing about Head & Shoulders being only suitable as a 'man shampoo', we had to eat our words when this left our hair soft and shiny and manageable.

Aussie Aussome Volume €

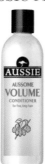

Great for adding socks to fine hair and it smells gorgeous too. Actually, you can't go wrong with most of the products in the Aussie range if you like their fresh and nourishing take. Three Minute Miracle is a cult conditioning product and is worth a try for stressed-out *gruaig*.

Vichy Dercos Technique Derma-Hair Care €

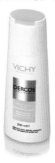

This is a range of seven specific shampoos that target common issues like dandruff, oily scalp, sensitivity and dry, damaged and brittle hair. One for everyone in the audience, basically, no matter your specific concern. If you haven't checked out these guys yet, give them a try. A bonus is that Vichy is so widely available here that you'll find it really easy to pick up.

Beaut.ienomics:
Dirty Tricks and
Smaller Sizes

Premium brands will do anything to protect their exclusive image and cutting prices is definitely not an option for them. Offers like three for two scream low-priced to them and they won't get on board with this kind of promotion – they see it as cheapening their brand.

So what do they do instead? Sales of some fancy salon products have been hit hard, but the profit hasn't fallen as you would expect.

Premium brands can be guilty of repackaging their products into smaller bottles. You look at a bottle of shampoo and think, 'Wow, that's cheaper than it was last year, I'll definitely buy that now.' But it's not cheaper at all – you're buying less product, so the price is exactly the same – or even worse, it may be more expensive.

Here's an example. Last year I bought a bottle of FancyPants salon shampoo for €20 and got 300ml for that price. This year I buy another bottle of FancyPants and it's only €18. Wow, I think, this has come down in price, and I'm delighted with my bargain. But I fail to notice that I'm only getting 250ml because of clever repackaging – and this means I'm actually paying more.

These amounts sound tiny, but do the multiplication and imagine thousands of people all paying a bit more. You are getting less product, are paying the same and the brands are protecting their profits. They're selling less product, but they're not making less money. The consumer, on the other hand, is being ripped off.

L'Oréal Professionel Shine Curl €€

Wild mops rejoice: this range is ace for controlling over-exuberant locks and taming frizz while still retaining curl. It has lots of nice ingredients like grapeseed extract and what the label refers to as 'shaping agents'. A read of the ingredients of course revealed that these agents were silicones, and boy do they work well here.

MorrocanOil Shampoo and Conditioner €€

These products were released like a movie tie-in based on the huge success of the original bottles of MorrocanOil. It broke box office records throughout the land for good reason and the spin-off range of shampoos, conditioners and styling products is just as good. Bear in mind that this is a salon range so it's not cheap, but it's very good. It's sulphate and phosphate free, kind to colour-treated hair and to top it off it's paraben free too, which means that they appeal across the board.

Make Your Own Hair Oil

Hair oils have taken the beauty world by storm and become incredibly popular. Shu Uemura, Orofluido, Joico, MoroccanOil, Avon and Kerastase have all launched hair oils promising to smooth and infuse hair with moisture and therefore cut blow-drying and styling time.

But the reality is that using oil to nourish hair is as old as … well, hair itself. Hot oil treatments have been around for yonks and kitchen cupboard oils like olive and coconut have been proven to penetrate the hair shaft. So if you don't feel like shelling out for a salon treatment, then heating up a couple of teaspoons of one of these oils and applying to dry hair can result in an instant moisture boost.

MoroccanOil or Moroccan Oil?

Everyone went crazy to try this treatment when it first became available. But here's the thing: there are two types of oil from Morocco. One is Moroccan Oil, the other is the salon preparation MoroccanOil (all one word). Confused? Here's the difference between them.

Moroccan Oil

This is argan oil and is the pure form of the oil, which is sourced in Morocco, often from Berber women's co-operatives. It's not the one that everyone got their knickers in a twist over and in its neat form can be used on the skin, so don't buy it by accident and lash it on your *gruaig* thinking it'll do the job of the product below.

MoroccanOil

This stuff works more like a serum than traditional conditioning oil. It does contain some argan oil, but is absolutely packed with silicones – and this is what does the job to smooth hair. Apply a couple of drops onto the palm of your hand and work through damp hair before blow-drying for a sleek result. MoroccanOil gives great shine and works well with curly hair too – those who love it absolutely swear by it for reducing styling and drying time and for making *gruaig* sleek. It isn't cheap though, and if you want to save, we would recommend good old John Frieda Frizz-Ease instead.

Permanent Blow-dry

The biggest hair trend of recent years (or ever) was permanent, 12-week and keratin hair treatments. They were subject to so much hype it was almost as if Jesus himself was walking the land once more. With a terrible dose of frizz and split ends, naturally: they weren't hot on conditioner in biblical times, so we're pretty sure if he ever does come back he'll be straight down to his local salon for a quick chemical fix.

Originating mostly in Brazil, Hershesons in London then flew the European flag for these hair straightening treatments and from there they came to Ireland, where we fell upon them with the kind of zeal that can only be mustered by those who are forced to endure the frizz we tend to suffer thanks to our maritime climate.

There's a lot of moisture in the air in Ireland and that means poufy, annoying, tangly hair. As a result, we're a perfect candidate for these sorts of treatments, but of course there had to be a complication.

12-Week Blow-dry

This one is also called the permanent blow-dry and it caused a veritable panic on the streets when it became available here. We read about all these great products that seem to be available in the US and South America years before we get them, so when they do arrive, it sparks a feeding frenzy.

Our big concern with the 12-week blow-dry — and every other treatment marketed as a long-term blow-dry — was the fact that most of them seem to contain formaldehyde. You know, *formaldehyde*, the potentially toxic and carcinogenic chemical that's used by embalmers and the like?

In order to make hair remain smooth and shiny throughout multiple washes and variations in weather, treatments like this need to be packed full of chemicals if they are to do their job.

Keratin Blow-dry

This is essentially a 12-week blow-dry masquerading as a conditioning treatment. It contains a chemical called aldehyde, which transforms into formaldehyde when exposed to high temperatures … like the ones produced during the treatment process.

Brazilian Blowout and Brazilian Blowout Zero

By the time this treatment arrived, Irish women were savvy about the formaldehyde issue, so we welcomed Brazilian Blowout with open arms because its selling point was that it was formaldehyde free. But it turned out that, er, it actually did contain formaldehyde and as a result it was banned in Ireland by the Irish Medicines Board. The company then developed Brazilian Blowout Zero, which contains no formaldehyde but instead uses glycolic acid to tame badly behaved hair. Does it work? Time will tell.

While some of these treatments disappointed us, what is true is that this sector of the hair market is improving all the time. We can expect to see lots more innovation, with new salon and home treatments that are safe and easy to use being developed. Hopefully we'll see prices come down too. The uncontrollably haired among us wait in hope.

John Frieda 3 Days Straight €

Fancy the thought of calming it all down for a few days and chasing the frizz away until your next shampoo – without having to shell out for a salon treatment? John Frieda 3 Days Straight might suit you down to the ground, then. Spray it on wet hair and the keratin-based solution wraps itself round hair strands that you then blow dry straight. Run it over with the straighteners and the sleek results will withstand humidity and frizzy conditions for three days.

Beaut.ienomics:
Touch Up Your Roots Yourself

Instead of hurrying to the hairdressers every time your dark roots threaten to blow your 'I'm a natural blonde' story out of the water, touch them up yourself. Covering greys and blending colours is much easier now with products like Nice'n Easy Perfect 10 available on the supermarket shelves. Many modern hair colours are formulated with no ammonia too, so there's no eye-watering stink either.

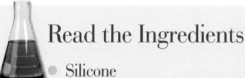

Read the Ingredients

Silicone

Anything that ends in 'cone' is a silicone (e.g. dimethicone). Silicone is often used in hair care and other cosmetics because it increases shine and slip, makes hair feel softer, conditions and reduces frizz.

So what's not to like? Well, some people aren't keen on it as an ingredient because they feel that it builds up on their hair and causes it to be limp and lacklustre. Claims are made that silicones 'suffocate' hair and produce a barrier between the hair and water.

This isn't necessarily true if you're just using a normal amount of product, but it's another one of those urban myths that abound in the cosmetic world. Silicones won't harm your hair and in fact they can be one of the most effective smoothing ingredients you can use if your hair likes them.

But if you feel the need for silicone liberation, try one of the silicone-free ranges from Phyto, Dr Hauschka and many other organic and natural cosmetic brands.

Hair Styling

We were smooth and sleek in the Noughties, but big hair is the trend that's taking us through the recession. The worse it gets, the bigger we might go. Irish hairdressers report that big hair is one of the most requested things from clients and we know why. It's nature, see: apes make themselves look bigger when facing adversity. Cats' tails turn into bottlebrushes and the hackles of dogs stand on end. It's biological power dressing – but we've replaced the shoulder pads with hairspray.

Big Hair
Recommendations

Babyliss Big Hair €€€€€+

This sold out everywhere last Christmas and it seriously couldn't be had for love nor money for weeks into February. The reason: it's really good and despite the name actually works on both thin hair with a tendency to flatness and also hair that's over-exuberant (by over-exuberant, we mean a frizzy mess when you try to do it yourself).

Use this when your hair is almost dry to brush volume into your roots and smooth down the length. As a friend of ours with a normally wild mane said, 'It's actually changed my life.' Can't say fairer than that, can you?

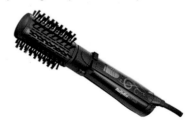

TLC Ceramic Hot Curling Brush €€

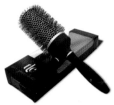

If you're already good at blow-drying, then this barrel brush is ideal for adding volume and creating nice, big, volume-tastic hair. Soft bristles and a ceramic coating that holds in the heat from the hairdryer longer means this gets the well-priced thumbs up.

Batiste €

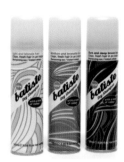

Batiste is a dry shampoo that basically works like a hair talc to soak up oil and freshen up your hair. It's great for getting another day or two out of your blow-dry, obviously, and the other thing this dry shampoo is good at is adding volume to limp locks. Once relegated to the bottom shelf at the chemist, Batiste has expanded its range and now comes in brunette, blonde and sparkly variations as well as loads of different smells. Other brands do their own versions, but Batiste is the cheapest and the best – you need a can of this stuff in your life.

Schwarzkopf OSiS Dust It Mattifying Hair Powder €€

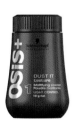

Like Batiste on steroids, this little red container bears a strong resemblance to a pepper pot stuffed with magic dust. Sprinkle a little throughout hair and you'll get instant volume and thickness, together with great hold. You won't need to use hairspray, so it's perfect for updos and creating a messy bedhead look too.

Schwarzkopf OSiS Body Me €€

Is it fair to give one range two picks? Yes, when they're as good as this one!
We've got a lot of love for the OSiS range. This product is fantastic for adding
stupendous root lift – just add it before you start your blow-dry.

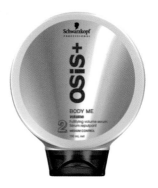

Blow Dry Root to Tip

Get extra volume by tipping your hair upside down for part of the blow-
drying process. When hair's still slightly damp, whip your locks towards
the floor and aim the heat at the roots. This forces the hair to dry
against the grain, which results in some much-appreciated root lift for
you.

Curly Hair

Curly hair requires a special type of product to control it and enhance its natural gorgeousness. Finding something with enough hold but which still allows flexibility in the curl is no easy task — and curly girls know that this task is a challenge of momentous proportion. There are tons of products out there optimistically called 'curl creams', but some of them are no good. These products get a lot of love — give one of them a go if you're at the end of your tether. Oh, and did we mention no crunchiness is tolerated? Good. Then we're on the same page.

- Aveda Be Curly €€€
- Trevor Sorbie Beautiful Curls Cream €
- Boots Essential Curl Crème €

Strengthen Serum with Conditioner

A bit of hair gel or conditioner mixed in with your serum or curl cream will give it more socks.

Rough and Texturised

Not everyone wants super-sleek groomed locks, and beach/bedhead hair is a big trend too: if you want that California surfer girl look, then check these out.

Recommendations

Matt Stylee: My Big Fat Texturised Hair Super Spray €€

Hairspray, wax spray and sea salt spray all in one – this super slush will turn into a spray when you shake it. Spray it all over to give messy surfer locks or just use it in the roots for a big lift. Work it through dry hair for a matte look 'do that won't move.

Umberto Giannini Glam Hair Grunge Glamour Tousled Salt Spray €€

Another good one for adding to that messed-up, just-fell-out-of-bed-looking-incredibly-sexy vibe. This gives a matte, lived-in result.

Paste and Putty

Short-haired types often use paste and putty to add a bit of control to hair. Putty is often really hard and inflexible, so scoop out a small amount and warm it in the palms of your hands. Once it begins to warm up and melt, it's ready for use. Lightly apply to hair using your palms and then style as required.

Smooth and Sleek

Hair serum is like manna from heaven for anyone prone to frizz and flyaways. Unless you're a hairdresser or very proficient with a hairdryer, you're going to need a bit of help to sleekify your hair. Try one of these great serums.

- Paul Mitchell Super Skinny Serum **€€€**
- Boots Botanics Serum **€**
- Lush R&B Revive & Balance Hair Moisturizer **€€**

Recommendations

Cult Product: John Frieda Frizz-Ease Hair Serum €

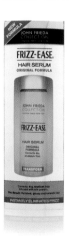

This stuff has been around for absolute yonks and is a bestseller for a reason. There are tons of varieties and you're guaranteed to find one to suit your particular source of hair trauma. It works really well to tame tresses and smooth even the most unruly of mops. Silicone is the star ingredient here and it's what performs the sleekifying magic.

The John Frieda range is sort of midway between a salon range and a supermarket brand. It includes shampoos and conditioners as well as serums, creams, mousses and wax — you name it, they've got it. Even better, you can usually pick up your favourites on special offer — three for two is a favourite promotion of this brand, so much so that we haven't paid full price for a bottle of Frizz-Ease for years. Result.

Using Serum

The key with serum is to use only a very small amount. If you lash on too much, hair will look lank and greasy. Apply just a drop or two into the palm of your hand and rub your hands together. Now lightly brush your hands down the length of your hair to tamp down pesky flyaways and tame frizzy ends. Oils are also great for anyone who's a slave to serum (see p. 123).

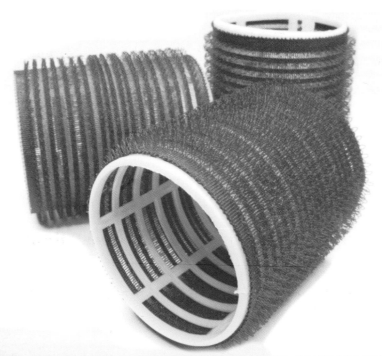

Hairspray

An oldie but such a goodie, we love hairspray for lots of reasons: it takes pen marks off patent leather, we've heard reports that people use it to set make-up (definitely not one to try at home) and of course you can lash it into your *gruaig* too.

We know hairspray has a bit of an old-fashioned vibe about it, but it's one of the most versatile and reliable styling products there is. Use it as a styling product as you blow-dry and of course to set your finished 'do as well. You can shell out for fancy-pants versions from brands like Shu Uemura if you like, but there's no need. You'll be able to pick up something affordable and really effective in your local chemist or supermarket. Here are two we like.

Recommendations

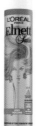

L'Oréal Paris Elnett €

We're fond of debunking the hysteria around cult products if we think they don't deserve the hype, but Elnett is a genuinely good product and a bestseller for a reason. Now available in a couple of different types, it's a light spray that won't soak the hair or leave it feeling crunchy. It gives good hold and brushes out with no gacky dandruff-style residue.

Garnier Fructis Style Bamboo Flexihold Shine and Hold Hairspray €

A bit more heavy duty than Elnett, this has good hold and gives a nice gloss to the finished result.

Give Hairspray Oomph with Mousse

If you've got very thick hair, a fine hairspray won't be enough to hold it solo. Either look for a heavy-duty spray (Aveda's Pure Abundance is a good bet) or make sure you prep hair for firm hold from the get-go with some heavy-duty mousse or thickefiers, then use your firm-hold hairspray as a final fix.

Beaut.ienomics: Thumbs Down for Travel Sizes

This is another area where premium brands pull a fast one with the downsized bottles that are actually much more expensive than a bigger size. They call them 'travel sizes' or 'minis' and by doing so you actually expect to pay more for less product. We've been trained to expect that smaller sizes will cost more, so we will pay well over the odds for a little trial kit with a couple of 15ml bottles of product. Clever, eh?

Budget brands are in on the game too, especially since the 100ml airline restrictions were introduced. Next time you fly, browse the rapidly expanding rack of travel-sized products in the airport pharmacy and be amazed at what they want you to pay for a weeny bottle of product. Save your cash – buy the big bottle and some inexpensive empty bottles that you can pick up in Boots or Marks & Spencer and decant enough for your holidays. Go splits with a friend if you're just trying something for the first time and aren't sure if you'll like it.

Start Duping and Save Money

Duping FAQs

- ### What's a dupe?

  In beauty blog parlance, a dupe is short for duplicate and it means a similar version of a high-end product at a much cheaper price. It can also mean two shades that are virtually identical, so it can stop you from spending money on three blushers that are indistinguishable.

- ### Er, surely no one buys dupes of stuff they already have?

  Unfortunately, we all do – and it costs us a fortune over time. We have a tendency to be attracted to the same shades over and over again, which explains why we have make-up bags full of pink and purple eyeshadows, all exactly the same. So many things influence our decision to buy a product – it might be brand new and everyone is talking about it, or it might just be that we've fallen in love with the packaging, or maybe we just really want to try out something from this particular brand. To stop yourself from accidentally buying a dupe of a shade you already have, ask yourself when you're about to make a purchase if you already have this exact shade. Chances are, you do.

- ## But surely the premium brands have better-quality stuff, so why would I buy a cheaper version?

Less-expensive brands have really upped their game and are now providing great-quality make-up with good pigmentation and lasting power. Sometimes you can get a virtually indistinguishable shade match at a fraction of the price.

The quality does tend to be better with more expensive brands, there's no doubt about it. You may find the products last longer and wear better on the skin. But if you're just dying to try out a new colour to see if it suits you or simply can't afford to stock up on endless Bobbi Brown palettes (like most of us), then it's a good bet you'll be able to find a cheaper version of it somewhere in the beautyverse.

Duping is the ultimate clever trick for the make-up junkie and means you can follow all the latest trends for a fraction of the price. Of course, all of this pales into insignificance if you love your premium brands like your MAC or NARS and are prepared to pay more for them. But even you can save money by making sure you don't accidentally buy a shade you already have. MAC in particular are really clever about churning out limited edition collections on a regular basis that people buy essentially for the packaging and so are more likely to pick up duplicate shades – especially as MAC often re-promotes shades you may have previously picked up.

Penneys copies catwalk fashion trends and more expensive collections while they're practically still on the runway and the cosmetic houses are no different. As soon as Chanel brings out its must-have nail varnish for the season, Barry M and Models Own will be feverishly beavering away to bring as close a shade match as they can to a chemist near you. (And a word to the wise: sometimes you're better off with those Chanel dupes. Fabulous as the colours may be, the formulation of Chanel varnishes just doesn't last and chips really quickly.)

So let's have a look at some of the most popular make-up products out there and the cheaper versions of them.

We like to make smart swaps where we can (more money for handbags, so) and our beauty bags are jammers with these clever buys.

Recommendations

NARS Orgasm Blush €€€ vs. e.l.f. Candid Coral Blush €

This is one of the best ways to try out a coral blush on the cheap. NARS's Orgasm is fiendishly priced, and while e.l.f.'s cheapo version can't hold a candle to the rubberised packaging of its more expensive doppelganger and it's nowhere near as silky-smooth to the touch, we challenge anyone to tell the difference on the face.

MAC Lipstick in Ruby Woo €€ vs. Rimmel Colour Show Off in Red Fever €

Ruby Woo is the classic matte red lippy. Not everyone is near a MAC counter or happy to pay the brand's prices, so how about a few quid for Rimmel's Colour Show Off in Red Fever instead? The shades aren't a precise match but the finish is retro-fab and longevity is great.

Benefit Posietint €€€ vs. 2True Cheek 'n' Lip Tint €

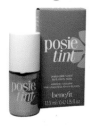 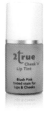

A brilliant dupe for Benefit's way pricier Posietint, 2True's Cheek 'n' Lip Tint is a tiny price and performs really well. We're seriously impressed, but do note it's better on cheeks than lips.

MAC Studio Fix Fluid Foundation €€€ vs. Revlon ColorStay Makeup €€

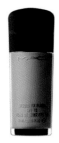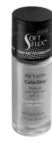

Studio Fix is one of MAC's eternal stars, giving great coverage, a soft finish and a big shade range. Offering it serious competition is Revlon's ColorStay Makeup, which gives a remarkably similar result in lots of shades, yet offers something MAC doesn't – ColourStay comes in versions for normal to dry skin and combination to oily. Very smart.

Lancôme Eyeshadow in Erika F €€€ vs. Gosh Trio Eyeshadow TR13 €€

Silvery, olivey and absolutely gorgeous, Erika F is a shadow that will suit all skin tones and eye colours. Sheer it out for day or lash it on for night, it's a stand-out neutral. Get the same look from Gosh Trio TR13, which happily contains two other shades you'll love as well.

Yves Saint Laurent Touche Éclat €€€€ vs. Aldi Lacura Beauty Concealer Pen €

Hands up – who hasn't tried Touche Éclat? Yup, that's all of us so. Get the look for a whole lot less at budget supermarket Aldi, as their Lacura Beauty Concealer Pen is a damn good substitute for the much pricier YSL.

Chanel Le Vernis in Paradoxal €€€ vs. Models Own Purple Grey €

None of us can resist Chanel's polish colours, but plenty can resist the prices. So instead of splashing out on Paradoxal, buy Models Own Purple Grey instead. Honestly – it's identical.

MAC Blacktrack Fluidline Eyeliner Gel €€ vs. Maybelline Eye Studio Lasting Drama Gel Eyeliner €€

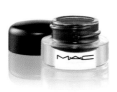

For too long it was impossible to get a good gel liner down the budget end of the market and MAC and Bobbi Brown held (expensive) sway. Now? Swap your MAC Blacktrack for Maybelline's fab Eye Studio liner and the best bit is you get an identical look and a really good little brush too.

Clinique Take the Day Off Makeup Remover for Lids, Lashes & Lips €€€ vs. Johnson's Daily Essentials Gentle Eye Make-up Remover €

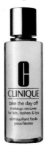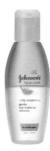

Both are dual-phase cleansers that you shake to mix and they make short work of eye make-up. It's always good to have one of these on hand for those super-stubborn smoky eye moments and we plump for Johnson's because it does the same job as Clinique but at a fraction of the price.

Make Up For Ever Mist & Fix €€€€ vs. e.l.f. Studio Makeup Mist & Set €

If you're a fan of make-up setting sprays – which are essentially water and a few other ingredients – then there's really not a lot of point in shelling out big bucks. Ditch the Make Up For Ever Mist & Fix habit and invest in some e.l.f. Studio Makeup Mist & Set instead.

Best Brands for Duping

In all honesty, budget and supermarket beauty is so good and the choice so wide these days that you could probably avoid department store counters altogether. Of course that'd be no fun – who doesn't enjoy those occasional luxe spends which look so fab on your dressing table? But if you do want to make a few conscientious swaps and save some cash, take a look at these brands.

Beaut.ienomics: Buyer Beware

When you do decide to dip your toes into the world of duping, just bear in mind that if you're switching to a cheaper brand, you may get the shade right but you may not get the lasting power, the finish or the intensity of pigmentation you get with the more expensive version.

Models Own

This brand came out of nowhere and soon became our number one source for Chanel polish dupes. If Uncle Karl Lagerfeld OKs it, Models Own copies it in about two seconds flat. A professional-style thin formulation means these polishes layer like a dream. They're decently priced, wear well and you're absolutely spoiled for choice when it comes to shades. We dare you to buy just one.

Catrice

Redesigned and fabulised, this German brand is frumpy no more. Its amazing prices belie the quality and quantity of products on offer. Fancy trying a lash growth serum that other brands sell for megabucks? No problem, and it'll just be a few quid. There are Urban Decay-alike brow kits, marbelised copies of MAC's Mineralize Skinfinish powders, more bright eyeshadow than you can shake a stick at and quality creamy lipsticks that offer the same finish as much more expensive bullets. Nails are another strong point for Catrice and it offers really good on-trend colours.

Gosh

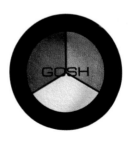

While it's pricier than Catrice, Gosh is another one to look at if you're in the market for a dupe or five. Of particular note are the Extreme Art Eye Liners that mimic MAC's more expensive Liquidlast offerings. Bonus? Gosh has a much better shade range than its pricier counterpart. Also check out the Velvet Touch Foundation Primer, which is a good approximation of Smashbox's cult Photo Finish product, and the Velvet Touch Eyeliners are also a dupe for MAC's Powerpoint pencils.

Inglot

Irish girls love, love, love MAC, but who wants to pay over the odds for a single shadow in a bonkers shade you won't wear much? Eh, no one, so that's why we recommend Inglot and in particular their really affordable Freedom System palettes. You choose the shades you want and you can buy the palettes in two, four, five and 10 pan options, meaning you can really tailor your choice to suit your pocket. Inglot is also great for affordable brushes, brilliant blush and more bright colours than you can shake a stick at.

Barry M

Another brilliant brand for whipping out nail polish dupes quick smart, we love Barry M for their fun colours, affordable prices and regular injections of fab fashion-forward shades. Plus Barry M's Dazzle Dust contains many similar shades to MAC's much pricier pigments.

2True

Find this little beauty company at Superdrug, where it seems to have carved a niche for itself paying homage to the works of Benefit. There are cheapo dupes for Benefit's boxed powders and tints and all for very little money. Well worth taking a look at.

Sigma and Crown Brushes

To get the best out of all your beauty bits (dupes or otherwise), you do need a few decent brushes. But they can be extremely expensive, so we recommend you look online. Sigma (www.sigmabeauty.com) offers dupes for MAC's make-up brushes and even uses the same numbering system, making your choice a cinch. Personally, Beaut.ie is fond of Crown Brushes (www.crownbrush.co.uk), who offers brilliant brush kits for very good prices. We've had our Crown brushes for years and can hand-on-heart attest to their quality.

Sleek

Another brand only available to us in Ireland over the Internet (but lucky Northern Irish gals can buy in Superdrug), everyone needs to own one of Sleek's great i-Divine shadow palettes. Sleek mimics the quality of much more expensive brands but at really affordable prices. Available in lots of colourways, the palettes contain 12 well-pigmented shadows in a mix of finishes, from mattes to shimmers.

e.l.f.

e.l.f., or Eyes Lips Face, to give it its proper moniker, is an online retailer that sells absolutely tons of products for tiny prices. Their slightly more expensive Studio line has some half-decent NARS dupes, like the aforementioned Candid Coral blush, and in the regular line look at the Benefit High Beam-alike Shimmering Facial Whip, while the All Over Colour Sticks are kinda sorta like NARS's Multiples.

Essence

Known as Catrice's little sister, Essence is another brand well worth checking out for the nail obsessed. They do loads of different types, sizes and finishes of lacquer, which allows you to mimic the shades available from much more expensive brands. Brilliant.

Beaut.ienomics:
Supermarket
Beauty Buying

The supermarket is fast becoming the place where most of us pick up day-to-day beauty products like cleanser, shower gel and body lotion. The bigger Boots stores and large chemists act like supermarkets too, with the same sales mechanisms and merchandising. They all have the same principles – pile 'em high, sell 'em cheap – and are great for big mass market brands.

One thing that the supermarkets excel at is own brand beauty. The standard is really high and ranges will copy competitors' products, blatently rip them off and present you with a very close copy indeed. Ingredients are replicated, packaging is replicated and to be honest a blind man on a galloping horse (as Beaut.ie Dad would say) would be hard pushed to tell the difference.

Look out for Tesco Skin Wisdom products, the Aldi Lacura range and some of the gems from the Marks & Spencer range – the Tess Daly collection is particularly good.

Features of Supermarket Shopping

- Three for two
- Buy one get one free
- 50 per cent extra free
- New products at introductory prices
- Buy this, get a teeny one of something else taped to the side
- Before a product relaunches in new packaging, it's often sold at a good discount.
- New packaging for old products
- Extra points or money off for special occasions or events (think Mother's Day, for example)

You'd be mad to turn up your nose at supermarket beauty product possibilities – they can save you a fortune.

Notes

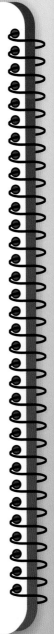

Notes

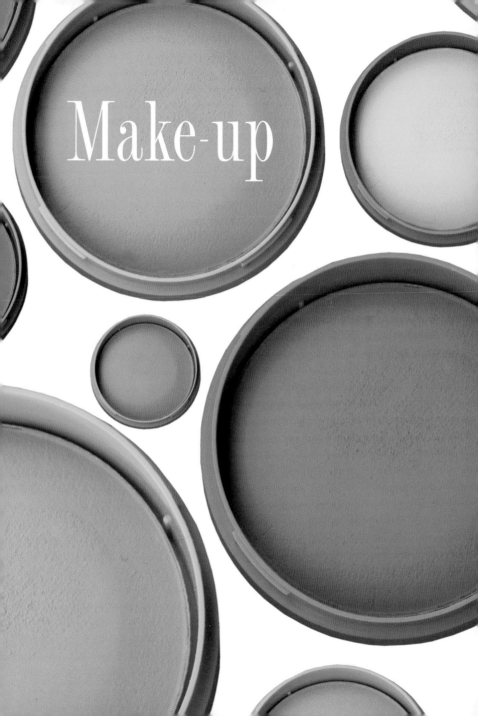

Make-up

Primer

No one had ever heard of make-up primer until a few years ago and boy, did we find out what we were missing when we finally invested. Now brands big and small produce primers for face, eyes and even lips, so we're spoiled for choice and can make sure our money goes further. Primer has an almost alchemical effect on skin and make-up and can really help to make your skin look smoother and give a key to make-up so that it sticks about for longer. With so many on the market, what do we rate?

Recommendations

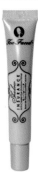

Shop Smart:
Too Faced Shadow Insurance €€

The squeezy, fluid texture of this makes it really easy to apply and blend, locking colour into place. Bonus? It can also be used as a mixing medium so that you can turn pigment powders into cream shadows. The tube lasts and lasts too.

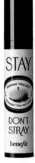

Benefit Stay Don't Stray €€€

A hybrid concealer-cum-primer, this is designed for use all around the eye area, so you dot it on above and below and then blend. It does conceal dark circles and acts as a key, clinging onto eyeshadow and locking it down for the whole day.

Gosh Velvet Touch Eye Primer €€

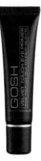

This isn't as silicone based as face primers are, so it's a good pick for eyes, sealing shadow in place. If you've got an oily complexion, get an eye primer in your life.

Penneys The Prime of Your Life €

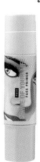

While this won't necessarily make foundation stick around longer, this suspiciously Benefit-alike tube will give you a smooth canvas on which to work and the pink colour of the product gives a bit of a brightening effect too. For the price, definitely worth a punt.

Urban Decay Primer Potion in Sin €€

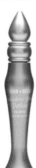

Another classic, this now comes in a couple of new colours, and Sin, a Champagne-shaded one, is a great bet for adding extra bling and shine to shimmer shadows. It ramps up shine and is a great bet for evening eyes.

L'Oréal Paris Studio Secrets Smoothing Resurfacing Primer €€

A decent dupe for Clarins's lovely Instant Smooth Perfecting Touch, it's also a good bit cheaper, which we like. Pop a little on across your nose and any open pores to give a nice base for foundation.

Maybelline Instant Anti-Age The Smoother Skin Retexturizing Primer €€

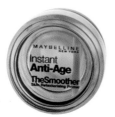

A good dupe for Smashbox's much pricier primer, Maybelline's version comes in a pot for easy access. It's got a nice firm texture and a little will fill in pores and fine lines.

Cult Product: Smashbox Photo Finish Foundation Primer €€€

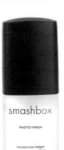

An oldie but such a goodie: this is a silicone-based primer that you apply under foundation and it fills in pores, lines and crags to give you a really smooth base for anything else you might like to throw on top. Pricey, but you need very little each time so it should last and last.

Don't Overuse Primer

Should you wear a primer every day? We say no. They're not generally necessary unless your skin is very sebum prone. It's not a great idea to overload the skin on a regular basis either. We tend to keep our foundation and eye primers for big nights out and special occasions. Bonus? We then amaze people with our line- and pore-free appearance to boot. Score!

Brush with Brilliance

Use your fingers when it comes to primers. You can use a paint brush-style foundation brush, like Estée Lauder's lovely one, but generally we don't bother. As these products tend to be packed with silicone and are transparent, it's easier to judge with fingers exactly where you're putting them.

Foundation

Let's get down to base matters: foundation is the one thing it's really essential to get right because it's the canvas onto which you'll literally be painting your other products. As a result, we tend to advise you spend a little more here because it's such a fundamental beauty buy.

Posher base often has better shade choices, formulation and longevity, but that's not to say there aren't fab products down the other end of the market too, because there are. Brands like Bourjois, Maybelline, Revlon and Max Factor in particular are well worth checking out if you're not in the humour to spend a lot of money.

Are You Pink or Yellow?

MAC foundations come in two shade families. NW is for pink-toned skins and NC is for yellow-toned. Bobbi Brown foundations are always yellow toned, so if you have pink-toned skin you are never going to get along with them without looking like something out of *The Simpsons*.

An easy way to work out if you're pink or yellow is to check your skin tone – if you've got sallow skin, you're yellow. Most Irish people are pink, so bear this in mind when you go shopping.

Beaut.ienomics: Discounting

You won't often see discounting with foundation unless it's a product that's being discontinued, but there are ways to get it more cheaply.

● Gift with Purchase

This is a great time to buy a premium foundation because you'll get some nice goodies in a cute make-up bag as an incentive. You often find that you'll get a trial version of a new foundation around the time it launches. Estée Lauder, Clarins and Clinique are all good for this.

● Introductory Offers

When a foundation is launched onto the market, particularly in the case of a budget product, the manufacturers want to make sure you try it and buy it. There will be all sorts of offers to lure you in, so if you're in the market for a new foundation, this is the time to buy.

● Sample

Make sure you get a sample of the foundation no matter what the price range. Samples in magazines and testers on the stand will give you an idea of texture and coverage and the pack information should indicate what type of skin the foundation is best suited to. Estée Lauder runs a service whereby they'll match your skin and shade and give you a free trial pack so you can check it out at home before you hand over your Laser card.

Recommendations

Shop Smart: Maybelline Dream Creamy Foundation and Maybelline Dream Satin Liquid €€

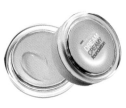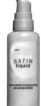

We reckon Maybelline does the best budget foundations, and while we'd like to see more shade choices, both of these products in the Dream range are very good. Choose the liquid for medium to full coverage and the compact version is great for on the go. Ditch the sponge though and use a brush.

Bourjois Healthy Mix Foundation €€

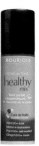

Great for normal to dry skins, this gives a nice glow on the skin, provides medium coverage and comes in a good shade range, with decent pale options. This is one of our favourites for day and it smells delicious too.

L'Oréal Paris Matte Morphose €€

Best mousse formulation we've used. This is a good bet for young, oily skin that needs coverage and oil control.

La Roche-Posay Toleriane Teint Mineral Compact €€€

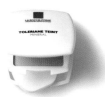

Great coverage and shine control plus skin-kind benefits are what makes this great. This is a great range for those with sensitive and reactive skins and it's also handy for carrying about and for touch-ups during the day.

Estée Lauder DoubleWear Light Stay-in-Place Makeup €€€€

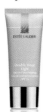

A brilliant old reliable, this lighter version of the classic DoubleWear foundation gives great coverage and oil control but isn't as heavy feeling on the skin.

Clarins Everlasting Foundation €€€

A new-generation long-wear foundation, we like this because it's well priced for a high-end brand and uses special porcelain pigments to offer lots of coverage but very little weight.

NARS Sheer Glow €€€€

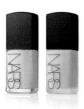

A really gorgeous foundation that will suit combination to normal skin. If you have a dry complexion, moisturise well beforehand. This blends and spreads like a dream, has great pale shades and gives a beautiful result. We save this one for night.

Diorskin Nude €€€€€

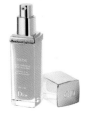

Another old favourite that dry skins and those up to a combination type will get along with, this provides nice coverage, comes in a good range of shades and is just very reliable altogether.

Max Factor Xperience Weightless Foundation €€

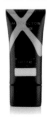

An impressive skin flatterer. For good skin days,* it gives a sheer finish that looks dewy, glowy and really healthy. Try this if skin is dry and dull.

* A good skin day: A day when everything is behaving itself. No mad breakouts or dry patches mean you can get away with a lighter foundation.

Chanel Vitalumière Aqua €€€€

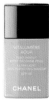

This is scrummy: light, dewy and creamy, it's nice to use and makes skin look and feel fab. If we had any gripe, it would be that the shade choice isn't the best, but this gives one of the nicest 'real skin' finishes we've seen. Quite sheer, it's best for good skin days.

MAC Studio Fix Fluid €€€€

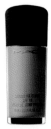

We always have a bottle of this old reliable on hand. It's a real workhorse product that performs. Providing good coverage, it comes in an absolute ton of shade options and is a good pick for those with normal to combination skin.

Giorgio Armani Lasting Silk UV €€€€€

One of our favourite glowy foundations, this is pricey but well named. It provides a gorgeous finish that's quite sheer and is a good bet for those with drier skin types. It evens out skin nicely and gives a wash of coverage, so it's brilliant for those days when you don't want to look too made-up.

Vichy Dermablend Foundation Cream Stick €€€

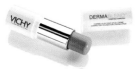

The ultimate in heavy coverage, this is excellent for those with serious camouflage needs and can be used to mask tattoos, port wine stains, rosacea and a whole load more.

Cult Product: Revlon ColorStay Foundation €€€

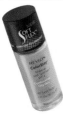

Available in versions for dry to normal and combination to oily, this is one of the best pharmacy foundation options and gets a lot of love in the beauty blogosphere. It's got a good shade range and provides medium to full coverage.

Brush with Brilliance

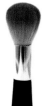

There's no need to splurge on a foundation brush if you don't want to – fingers will generally do the job fine, but for special occasions or to build coverage, a brush can be really helpful. We've got two we like a lot. MAC's 187 Duo Fibre Brush buffs on liquid base perfectly. Or try a more traditional paintbrush-style tool: EcoTools Bamboo Foundation Brush is a good bet. Its synthetic bristles are ideal, as they don't soak up too much product and it won't break the bank either.

Foundation Facts

● Touch of Foundation

Products claiming to have 'a touch of foundation' are basically just a marketing ploy: they're tinted moisturiser. Don't be fooled if you're looking for a lot of coverage – you won't get it here. For good skin days though, they're absolutely grand.

● How to Shade Match

Keep the mantra in your head that you must not pick too dark a shade. Repeat a hundred times: I am not an orange and my foundation must be the same colour as my skin. Test foundation by applying a little along your (make-up free) jaw line – it should blend in perfectly. If it doesn't, try another shade or two. If we see any of you looking like a satsuma, we'll be handing out lines.

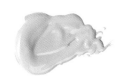

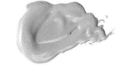

● Warming Yourself Up

The main reason a lot of Irish gals wear the wrong shade is they want to look like they have a little colour on the skin. But this is the wrong way to go about it – if you're worried about looking too pale, you can warm up with blusher or bronzer. Make sure you only apply it to the high points of the face, or basically the bits that would naturally be kissed by the sun.

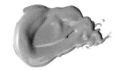

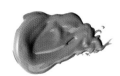

Beaut.ienomics:
Foundation Trend:
Take Two

One trend that we've noticed is the increasing popularity of people either downgrading their foundation to a less expensive brand or buying two brands of foundation – one for everyday and one for 'good'. Diehard Dior fans might have switched to Maybelline for trips to the shops and the school run, while others are simply mixing their foundation with a bit of moisturiser to eke it out.

If you're feeling the pinch, this is a great move, as foundation is probably one of the most expensive products you shell out for on a regular basis.

Recommendations

Get Your Rocks Off with Mineral Make-up

This is a craze that's still going strong, and while we're not that enamoured with mineral powder foundation, we know lots of you are. Having tried a lot of what's out there, we think this make-up works best if you've got oily skin.

If you're fed up with foundation sliding off your face a couple of hours after you've applied it, then it's time to give mineral powder a try. It literally — and this is gross — soaks up the oil. Dry and dehydrated types often find it actually accentuates their scaly bits and fine lines, so we say avoid it.

But now that everyone and their granny have brought out mineral ranges, here's a quick list of three of the big sellers to help you to decide who to buy from.

Bare Minerals

The granddaddy and originator of the craze, Bare Minerals continues to hold its majority and has recently expanded into skincare too. There's absolutely tons of choice in this line-up and lots of fun products too.

Everyday Minerals

These guys sell online and allow you to buy inexpensive sample packs that are cost effective and give you the chance to see if this stuff will work for you before you lay out the big bucks.

Lily Lolo

Another company that started life online, Lily Lolo can now be bought in some retailers too. Lots of choice, pure mineral formulations and some nice little shadows and blushers make this one popular.

Concealer

Concealer is a tricky beast that comes in many guises. There's the camouflaging cover-up that will hide blemishes and dark circles because it contains lots of lovely pigment and there are highlighting concealers that are lightweight and work by reflecting light and adding radiance. Then there's the choice between paste, cream or fluid, pot, pen or stick. Is it any wonder we're confused? Not to worry, we've sorted the wheat from the chaff for you.

Cheap Concealers Work Just as Well as Pricey Ones

Cheaper concealers can work just as well as pricey ones. Keep an open mind and follow the recommendations here – you might find your dream concealer in Tesco as easily as you'll find it at a department store.

Concealer FAQs

- ### Should I put on concealer first or last?
Apply your base and then have a look at yourself in the mirror. If things really need covering at that stage, then get to work. If you have a particularly Vesuvius-style zit to cover, do it before the foundation goes on.

- ### Are fingers fine?
Generally, yep, fingers do the trick nicely because they help to warm the product slightly and that in turn helps it to spread evenly. Use a patting motion to set the product in place.

If you'd rather use a brush, which is more hygienic, then look for one with synthetic bristles. There's no need to spend a fortune – you can buy really good synthetic brushes for a small outlay from brands like e.l.f. and EcoTools. And make sure you wash the brush regularly – nothing stinks like a manky concealer brush.

Recommendations

Shop Smart:
Barbara Daly Concealer for Tesco €

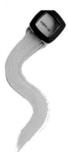

This is such an old reliable – if you find it, buy it. A little pot of super-duper pigmented goodness, nothing stands up to this powerhouse product. Dark circles are no match for it, spots run and hide and it's also good for covering up redness.

Benefit Erase Paste €€€

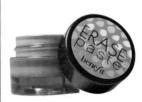

Benefit really does make some of the most fantastic matte cream concealers. Along with their cult product Boi-ing, this is a great concealer and will magic away even the reddest of spots with a wave of its tiny spatula. Great for use around the eye area too.

Penneys Ta Ta For Now €

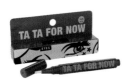

A surprise find in the Penneys beauty range, which all too often doesn't step up to the plate. But this is a great light-reflecting pen concealer that has good coverage and is as effective as the pricier picks it's aping. For a couple of euro we really can't find fault and it will work well with your pricier foundation.

Catrice Allround Concealer €

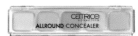

What's nice about this is that for a bargain basement price, this kit tackles colour correcting and camouflaging. You get three concealers and two corrective shades, which adds up to a very good kit for the money. Hide redness and yellow tones with the correctors and mix your own concealer shade from the three options. With roughly the same level of coverage as Touche Éclat, this gives a lightweight result.

Aldi Lacura Beauty Concealer Pen €

This is the famous supermarket concealer that's usually referred to as 'the Aldi Touche Éclat'. It does a good job of covering dark circles and brightening the eye area, blends really well and doesn't look cakey or settle into wrinkles.

Rimmel Stay Matte Dual Action Concealer €

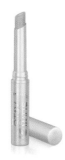

A good bet for those with oilier skin or those who are prone to spots, Stay Matte Dual Action Concealer has a treatment core that can help to speed up the healing of the zit it's hiding. Coverage is good and this feels quite dry to the touch, so it stays where it's put yet can be blended for a natural-looking finish.

Rimmel Match Perfection Concealer €

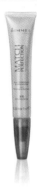

Match Perfection acts as an under-eye concealer and highlighter in one. Available in a brush-topped squeezy tube, it's apparently able to adapt to your skin tone. We're not so sure about that, but it's nice to use, covers dark circles well and doesn't make the delicate eye area feel dry and tight.

Cult Product: Bobbi Brown Creamy Concealer Kit €€€€

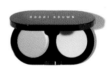

One of our long-time favourite concealing products, this is particularly good for use around the eye area. This stuff really is creamy. The pigmentation and coverage is great – use this at the inner corner of the eye by the nose, and ta dah! Instant lightening and brightening (and hopefully a few years off, too).

Beware Reverse Panda

Reverse Panda refers to someone who applied so much concealer that it turns the whole area around their eyes white under camera flash. Brigette Neilson is a member of the Reverse Panda species, as are Eva Longoria and Caprice (who's rumoured to use it all over her face). Reverse Panda is commonly accompanied by a Crime Against Fake Tan. Just think of a panda with orange fur and white circles around his eyes. You've got the picture now.

Blusher, Bronzer and Highlighter

We really love blusher and so will you if you've never used it before. Lots of women are scared of rouge and yes, it can seem a bit scary — after all, no one wants to look like Aunt Sally crossed with Bosco, or in fact any form of rosy-cheeked hybrid of the two.

But knowing what suits your skin tone and learning how to apply it can make all the difference to your overall look. Plus blusher can transport you from cadaver to cover girl in about two seconds flat — and really, what's not to love about that? As a result, we call it one of our true transformative products.

How to Apply Shimmer

Shimmer is beautiful and can really enliven a pale complexion, but too much can make skin look shiny and greasy. Go sparingly with this stuff and apply with a very light hand. We like to gently sweep some on at the top of cheekbones, on the temples and lightly down the nose. Cool-toned silvery highlighters flatter sallow-toned skin and golden-shaded products add lovely depth to cool skin tones.

Recommendations

Shop Smart: MAC Pigment in Vanilla €€€

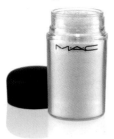

Why buy two products when you can buy one? A smart make-up artist trick is to make products multitask: you can triple up MAC's Vanilla Pigment as a shadow, brow highlight and facial luminiser. It looks great lightly buffed across the tops of cheekbones, on the temples and down the nose.

Essence Silky Touch Blush €

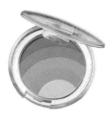

A pocket-money price and good shade choice make this a make-up bag must. The texture is the big surprise here: it's lovely and silky. Colour us impressed.

2True Cheek 'n' Lip Tint €

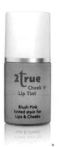

These budget cheek and lip tints dupe Benefit's much pricier Benetint and Posietint liquids. Definitely punching above the price point, these are loaded with pigment, can be worn sheer or built up for a serious pop of colour and have good lasting power.

e.l.f. Studio Blush €

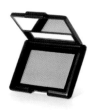

It seems you can't turn crookedy in the beautysphere without brands trying to knock off NARS. e.l.f.'s slightly pricier Studio line is one that's doing it pretty well. Studio Blush in Candid Coral is a good bet for blusher newbies, being well priced and quite sheer, so you can build colour gradually.

Tess Daly Beauty Face Glow €€

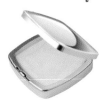

You get absolutely scads of this and it'll last forever. A cool-toned cream shimmer, it looks beautiful and can be applied everywhere: try it in the cupid's bow, on cheek and brow bones and even on shoulders and legs.

Prestige Skin Loving Minerals €€

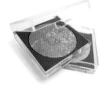

Modelled on MAC's cult Mineralize Skinfinish powders, Prestige's Skin Loving Minerals powders make lovely shimmery bronzers that give a golden glow to skin. Well priced, too.

Rimmel Sun Shimmer Bronzing Compact Powder €

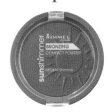

With mattes and shimmers and a couple of shade choices, Rimmel's Sun Shimmer bronzers are really good budget reliables. Use the mattes to contour and sculpt the face, while the shimmers can be used to give a lovely post-holiday glow.

The Balm Mary-Lou Manizer €€€

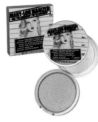

We're very glad this cute and quirky range is now more widely available in Ireland. Mary-Lou Manizer is a shimmery, oyster-coloured pressed powder that you can use lightly all over foundation to set it, or as a highlighter on the planes of the face where they catch the light.

Une Breezy Cheeks Blush €€

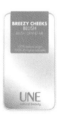

This eco-friendly brand from the peeps at Bourjois contains loads of skin-friendly products in nicely natural shades. This cream blusher applies really easily and looks flattering and soft on cheeks.

Cult Product: Benefit Coralista €€€€

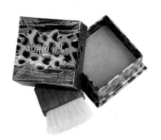

Move over NARS and yer Orgasm. There's a new cult must-have in town and it's definitely Benefit Coralista. This yummy-scented peachy wonder with subtle golden shimmer is incredibly flattering on pale *cailíns* and is far easier to find in Ireland than NARS too. Also check out Bella Bamba, a watermelon-toned newbie from Benefit that we're loving a lot too.

Bronze Basics

Much like highlighter, bronzer is not something you should ever use to colour in your whole face. If you do, you'll look weirdly flat and mucky. Bronzer should be applied very sparingly to the planes of the face that naturally catch the light, so you'll want to lightly buff it on the temples, cheeks, chin and nose. That way, you'll achieve a glow that looks natural and flattering. For most pale Irish gals, the lightest shade of bronzer in any range will be the most suitable. If you use bronzer to contour, keep it matte and not shimmery.

Which Blusher to Choose?

How to know what shade suits? If you have a lot of redness or colour in your cheeks, then give pink a miss and look for something peach or apricot toned instead.

Pale gals look great in coral tones and it suits dark-haired, pale-skinned girls just as well as sallow-skinned blondes. Darker-skinned girls can get away with really rich, pigmented colours, and brands like Sleek on the budget end and NARS on the luxe side of things offer deep reds, burgundies and bronzes that suit really well.

Picking a blusher with a small, subtle amount of sophisticated shimmer can add an extra dimension to your make-up and will catch the light as you move, giving a dewy finish to your make-up.

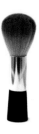

Brush with Brilliance

Our favourite blusher brush is one by Smashbox with an angled head. It's soft and fluffy and applies powder products perfectly. You can buy a similar brush from Crown Brushes that will do the job nicely. For cream and liquid blushers, we like Gosh's Light Weight Duo Fibre brush, which we also use for very pigmented powder rouge that threatens to turn us into Bosco.

Calming Down Overload

If you apply too much product, don't panic: you can either apply a little liquid foundation to a duo-fibre brush like MAC's 187 and gently buff it in to tone down the colour, or buff it out with some loose or pressed powder and a soft powder brush.

Lipstick and Lip Gloss

A nother really fun beauty bit, lipstick and gloss can instantly change your look and take you from frump to fab with the swish of a wand. In the battle of the lip products that's been raging since time immemorial, gloss has held sway in recent years and lipstick was firmly relegated to the frumpy bin. Not any more: stellar launches from king of cool Tom Ford and lovely new lines from Chanel, Yves Saint Laurent, Shiseido and Lancôme have brought this beauty staple back into the limelight. We're fans of both – it's twice the fun – so here are our top lip picks.

Top It Up

How do I make my lipstick last all day? Here's the bad news: you can't. Unless you sit still, not smiling, talking, eating or drinking, chances are you'll have to reapply at some point. Those women with eternally perfect-looking pouts? There's no secret – they just nip to the loo now and then for a judicious top-up.

Recommendations

Shop Smart: NYX Black Label Lipsticks €

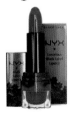

This is a brand you have to hunt for in Ireland, so we prefer to buy online. The Black Label Lipstick line is really affordable and contains over a hundred shades of creamy, opaque colours. Best of all, these are great dupes for Yves Saint Laurent's much more expensive Rouge Volupte lipsticks.

Rimmel Colour Show Off €

These are the best budget mattes we've found. While you need a little bit of balm underneath, these last and last, are a really affordable pocket-money price and come in great fashion-forward shades.

No7 High Shine Lip Gloss €€

It's a moisturising, juicy gloss that softens lips. Great over lipstick, as it doesn't have much colour itself.

Bourjois Rouge Hi-Tech Lip Tints €€

Lip tints are big business with lots of brands launching marker-style pens, but we have to fess up and say our hearts still belong to Bourjois. These tints come in great colours and have a soft applicator that makes use a cinch.

Karaja Crystal Gloss €€

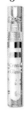

It can be really hard to find gloss with loads of colour payoff, so well done Karaja. The brand's a little under the radar but this delivers lots of colour and shine – just what we want.

L'Oréal Paris Glam Shine Reflexion Lip Gloss €€

A really good product for the price, with lots of colour, shine and importantly, it stays put for a lot longer than other brands we've trialled.

Maybelline Color Sensational Lipstick €

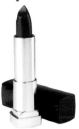

This lippy line is widely available nationwide, which is a great plus and it has some really good colours to boot. The Fatal Red shade is our pick - it's a good night-time matte.

Bourjois Sweet Kiss Lipstick €€

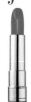

Lovely packaging, great shade choices and comfort are the boxes we tick with these yummy lippies, which have an old-fashioned scent of violets.

Revlon ColorBurst Lipstick €€

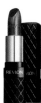

If you're not mad on the flat, matte look lipstick often has, then these lipsticks are a lovely pick. ColorBurst's formula is packed with pigment, but there's also lots of shine and they hang about on the lips a decent amount of time too.

Poppy King for No7 €€

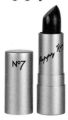

Creator of the cult Lipstick Queen line, Poppy King's collaboration with Boots is fab. Sheer lipsticks and glosses are a great way to get into lipstick without going for full-on opaque colour. Cute packaging is the icing on the cake.

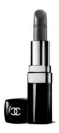

Cult Product:
Chanel Rouge Coco €€€

Let us count the ways we love this stuff: the double C logo, the quality of the formulation, the shades and the sheer handbag envy are all reasons to indulge. Oh, and did we mention the double C?

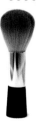

Brush with Brilliance

We're straight-from-the-tube or fingers gals when it comes to lipstick. Make-up artists often advise that lip brushes can help colour last longer, as it's pushed more effectively into the skin, but we can't say we've ever noticed a major difference.

Beaut.ienomics:
Airport Shopping

We're asked time and time again if it's really cheaper to shop in the airport. An unequivocal yes is the answer. The cosmetics on sale in The Loop in Dublin Airport are usually up to 25 per cent cheaper than the high street – and you can pick up an even better bargain if you look out for special offers.

David McWilliams was famously surprised to hear that the (tiny) MAC concession in Dublin Airport was the busiest in Europe, but we weren't. Every MAC addict knows that it would be sheer madness to walk past the MAC shop and not buy a few of your staple items, because the savings are that good.

Revenue from airport shopping is a hugely lucrative business for airport authorities. The first duty free in the world was opened in Shannon Airport in the 1950s and was such a success that this model was copied all over the world. Now, of course, duty-free doesn't operate unless you leave the EU, but airport shopping has nimbly stepped in to take its place. You don't think they created The Loop at Dublin Airport and spent millions on the design of the shopping facilities in Terminal 2 out of the goodness of their hearts, do you? Thought not.

You're trapped in a fiendishly clever purpose-built environment – a specially created impulse shopping paradise. All the fantastic shopping facilities are specifically designed to get you to spend – and here's how they do it.

The no man's land of the airport departure halls is an unfamiliar environment and you're out of your comfort zone. Plus you're about to take a journey to another unfamiliar environment. The whole experience is hugely unsettling, and whether you recognise it or not, your anxiety level is heightened. You're excited and maybe stressed – all perfect conditions to encourage impulse shopping behaviour.

And even worse: you're a captive audience. You couldn't get out of that departures limbo if your life depended on it. So there's nothing else for you to do while waiting for your flight but consume overpriced food – and consume all the fabulous premium goodies you see glittering on shelves around you.

Walk this way – designer sunglasses! Walk on a bit – the Jo Malone counter! And keep walking. God knows there's miles of walking in an airport. And cunningly, you must walk past rows and rows of shop fronts selling you books, fragrances, alcohol and giant Toblerones.

And the best bit for the airport: you can't bring anything back. Yes, that's right – when was the last time you ever 'brought something back' to the airport? There's no time to check your purchases properly, you're in a hurry and you've probably just grabbed them off the shelves anyway. So even if the purchase is unsuitable or the shade or size is wrong, you'll just put up with it. They've got us by the short and curlies and there ain't a damn thing we can do about it.

Eyeshadow

From pots of pigment and luxury palettes to solo shadows, the years have proven that no, a girl cannot have enough shimmering navy eyeshadows.

There's so much choice out there these days that you honestly don't need to go near a department store counter for your shadow fix unless you genuinely want to. This is one sector where budget really rules – here are our picks.

Recommendations

Shop Smart: Inglot Freedom System €€

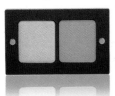

Terrific because you can choose the shades you want and build a palette full of colours that you'll actually use. Inglot's Freedom System is really well priced and the colour choice is second to none, with great pigment and finish choices. Completely brilliant.

Revlon ColorStay Eyeshadow Quads €€

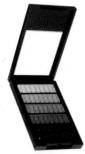

Not everyone wants to look like they've been attacked by the make-up gun and sometimes intense pigment isn't needed. A subtle finish is what a lot of women want, especially during the day, and these quads provide a sheer wash of satiny colour that's buildable.

Barry M Dazzle Dusts €

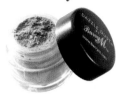

Ah, good old Barry and his Dazzle Dusts. They're only a few quid a pop and we dare you to get to the bottom of one of 'em. With lots of dupes in the range for MAC's much pricier Pigments, these loose powders are great value for money and a sure bet for anyone who likes a lot of shimmer and shine.

Dior 5-Colour Eyeshadow €€€€€+

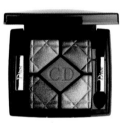

We really can't heap enough praise on these gorgeous yokes: Dior's 5-Colour Eyeshadow palettes come in a couple of different types (the Designer version has a cream liner included, for example), and while they're very much an investment buy, they're well worth it. You get five complimentary shades in each palette in a variety of finishes. Yum, we love 'em.

17 Solo Eyeshadows €

Completely brilliant for night-time drama. Great satin and metallic finishes, loads and loads of pigment and a creamy texture makes this shadow excellent for achieving a fab-looking smoky eye.

Sleek i-Divine Palettes €

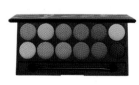

While you do have to buy these online, they're well worth it. Sleek has a range of 12 pan palettes that cost under a tenner and contain a really well-edited selection of shadows in matte and shimmer textures. There's a big mirror in the lid too, and while the supplied applicator is fairly crap, the shades definitely make up for it. We've got the Storm and Original i-Divines and highly recommend them.

L'Oréal Paris Colour Appeal Chrome Shine and Chrome Intensity €€

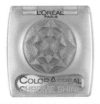

Delivering a proper blingin' shine, these metallic shadows really punch above their weight. Creamy and shimmery, they're gorgeous for night-time peepers and make a real impact on the lids.

Gosh Trio Eyeshadow €€

You get a lot of bang for your buck with Gosh's trio eyeshadows, which are very well priced. These come in tons of colourways too, so you're really spoiled for choice.

Make Up For Ever Aqua Cream €€€

These are the sort of things make-up artists lose their life over: for use all over the face, Aqua Creams definitely get most use on our eyes (we're not too into the green blusher look), and because they're properly waterproof they really stick about. With brilliant bright colours, these also act as a primer for powder shadow, helping it to last the day. Expensive, but these last a long time.

Max Factor Masterpiece Colour Precision Eyeshadow €

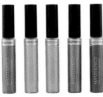

While the shade choice is a little limited, these are great for anyone who hates fiddling with powder shadow. Quick and simple to apply, they'll last all day too. The pink is particularly flattering and eye opening.

Cult Product: MAC Eyeshadows €€

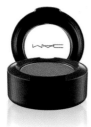

MAC's dominance in the make-up market is legendary and it's all thanks to a huge shade selection, loads of finish options and bazillions of limited edition collections. As a brand it's hard to beat for shadow choice, variety and sheer fun.

What Colour Will Suit You?

It can be hugely confusing to work out what will suit your eye colour. Grey, taupe and bone shades are a good bet for most eye colours, but let's get specific.

- **Green Eyes**

  Purples and pinks are flattering, as are plum-toned browns and burgundies. Deep forest greens can also help to brighten green eyes.

- **Blue Eyes**

  Russet, copper and orange-toned colours will really make blue eyes stand out. Peach and gold also suit and darker shades like blacks and grey work too.

- **Brown Eyes**

  Being on the opposite end of the colour spectrum to brown, blues can be a good bet. Navy makes hazel eyes look clear and bright and olives, greys and khaki will also flatter.

- **Grey Eyes**

  Dark shades can help to brighten the whites of the eye, helping the iris colour stand out. Purples work, as will Prussian blue, charcoal and deep brown tones.

Finishing Touches

What's up with shadow textures? It can be a bit baffling to be faced with a whole slew of different finishes. Here's what's what.

- **Matte**

  Revlon, MAC, Make Up For Ever and Inglot all have a good selection of mattes. These can be a bit hard to work with but have no shimmer or shine at all, so are good for day.

- **Glitter**

  Stand up, Urban Decay, the undisputed king of bling. This type of shadow is characterised by visible sparkle and glitter. Beware: they can be hard to wear and you'll often find fallout on your cheeks. Think about using a primer first.

- **Frost and Shimmer**

  Avoid if you have dry or crepey lids – highly shimmery or pearlised shadows will sit into and accentuate creases. Sleek and L'Oréal Paris make good shimmers and you'll know them by their sheeny finish.

- **Iridescent**

  This sort of shadow is duo-toned and looks different depending on the way the light's hitting it. Great for night-time eyes, iridescent shadows can also be layered over a black base for extra drama. Check out Accessorize's Illusion eyeshadow range for some good offerings.

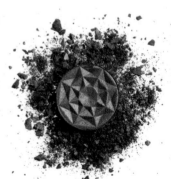

- **Satin**

  An easy shadow type to wear for most people, satins are halfway between a matte and a shimmer and give a nice sheen on the skin. Chanel's Ombres Contraste Duos are a great pick.

- Cream

These are liquid or cream textured and can be applied with the fingers. Use them solo or as a base for powder shadow. Check out Max Factor, Estée Lauder, MAC and Make Up For Ever, all of whom make great cream shadow products.

Blend, Blend, Blend

We're happy to use our fingers for foundation, concealer and even cream blush, but we're pretty evangelical about using brushes for eyeshadow. The fact is, you'll never get a fab-looking professional finish if you're messing about with crap sponge applicators and fingers. Neither is designed to do any of the jobs brushes do so well, like precise colour placement and blending. Blending is crucial for a good finish, so at the very least, try to buy a shadow brush and a blending brush. See below for some suggestions for what to buy.

What Are the Three Colours in Trios Meant For?

The pale shade is for using all over the lid, the middle colour can be used in the crease of the eye and the dark shade's for lining. Simple!

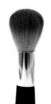

Brush with Brilliance

There's no need to spend the earth on eye brushes – try Crown Brush, which you can buy online. Their kits can be a great starting point for a brush newbie and they don't cost a fortune. e.l.f.'s Studio Line brushes are also worth a punt. Closer to home, check out Inglot's big range of well-priced tools, have a look in Boots for EcoTools and Marks & Spencer can be worth a look too.

Eyeliner

The cat's eye flick refuses to go out of fashion. The reason it's such a perennial favourite is because it's flattering, easy to achieve (once you've had a bit of practice) and there are absolutely tons of products on the market to help you achieve the look. Here are our favourites.

Joining the Dots

It can be hard to get the flick right if you're a novice, so a good trick is to place two or three dots across the lash line and then join them up to form a single, smooth shape. Eyeliner novices may also find a felt tip-style pen easier to use than a brush and cream product. Try placing the tip lengthwise along the lash line and literally press the product into place. A sneaky cheat – but an effective one!

Recommendations

Shop Smart: Maybelline Eye Studio Lasting Drama Gel Eyeliner €€

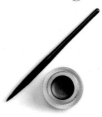

This is a brilliant buy: not only do you get a creamy gel liner, but you also get the brush, which is worth the price of the product all on its own. This little pot of goodness definitely competes with the big boys and gives MAC's Fluidlines and Bobbi Brown's Long-Wear Gel Eyeliners a serious run for their money.

Gosh Velvet Touch Eye Liner €

Dupes for MAC's Powerpoint Eye Pencils, Gosh's Velvet Touch Eye Liner pencils come in loads of great shades and stay where they're put. You can use them on the waterline too.

Rimmel Flash Eyeliner €

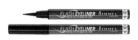

Fans of marker-style eyeliners will like this one. It's nicely black, doesn't drag across the lids and makes cat's flicks possible in mere seconds.

Gosh Extreme Art Eye Liner €€

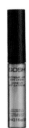

Proving they definitely keep a close watch on what's happening at MAC, Gosh's Extreme Art Eye Liners are a dead ringer for MAC's Liquidlast liners, except Gosh's come in way more shades. Longevity on these is amazing and they deliver a bright, plastic shine.

Bourjois Effet Smoky Pencil €

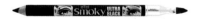

Our criteria for pencil liners is that they've got to be soft – there's nothing worse than dragging a hard nib across delicate lids. Hurray – Bourjois Effet Smoky Pencil is nicely smudgy and available in several shades. It's a really good basic kohl-style pencil to have in your kit, especially if rock chick eyes are your thing.

Prestige Total Intensity Eyeliner €

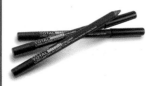

These are quite frankly brilliant value: super creamy and smooth, they're packed with colour and set to form a budge-proof finish. While you don't get a big shade choice, in terms of finish and intensity, they're a good dupe for Urban Decay's much more expensive 24/7 pencils.

Avon SuperSHOCK Gel Eyeliner €

We're really impressed with this super-smooth creamy gel pencil liner. It glides on, sets and stays all day because it sets a few seconds after application. Fab.

Cult Product: Bobbi Brown Long-Wear Gel Eyeliner €€€

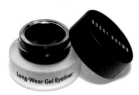

This is the gold standard when it comes to gel liner. It's absolutely fantastic. Creamy, smooth and deeply pigmented, it glides on and it will not budge until you decide you want it to. Pricey, but very definitely worth the spend.

Easy Fix

No one gets their make-up right all of the time – not even the pros – and liner's one of the hardest to get looking good. So honestly, don't fret if you make a mistake or it all looks a bit wonky – you can fix it. Keep some cotton buds on hand and use them to clean up jagged edges and tidy curves. It'll be our little secret.

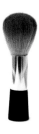

Brush with Brilliance

We're most partial to cream and gel liners that you apply with a brush. Smashbox's Arced Eyeliner Brush is a great pick, but we also love brushes with small, rounded tips, like Make Up For Ever's 3p brush, which came in a five-brush collection. It's a travel-sized lip brush, but it happens to be completely brilliant for applying eyeliner too.

Mascara

So many mascaras, so little time! There are zillions of mascaras out there, with new ones being launched onto the market almost weekly. It's a gladiatorial arena where only the strong survive and the weak get torn apart by the lions pretty quickly.

So what works really well? We think there are two things to consider here and they are gunk and wand. The wand should work like the best brassieres – to push lashes up, lift and separate. The difference must be immediate and instantly noticeable. The gunk needs to be dark and dramatic, stretchy, non-gloopy and it absolutely must not flake down our faces after two hours' wear.

So without further ado, here's what's great.

Beaut.ienomics: Gift with Purchase

It's an absolute mascara bonanza when it comes to gift with purchase freebies. A mini mascara (or full size if you're really lucky) is almost always included. Brands promote their new mascara lines with GWP promotions or use it as a chance to lure in new customers with cult mascara buys.

This is how we first tried Estée Lauder's Double Wear mascara and became so enamoured we continued to make many purchases of same. As well as being a great way to try something out, mini mascara is also great for the handbag.

Recommendations

Shop Smart:
Essence Stays On and On and On €

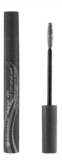

Cheap as the proverbial chips, this one: it's a really good pick for daytime eyes. We don't find it dramatic enough for night, but because it's so cheap, grab it for work and then spend a little more on something super-duper for going out. This will add definition and length and is a steal at the price.

Rimmel Max Bold Curves €

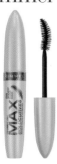

A good curved brush that pushes lashes up and into a curl, it's nicely black, doesn't clump and can be built and built for some serious volume. One of the best bargain mascaras for night we've found for quite some time.

NARS Larger Than Life Volumizing Mascara €€€

This is expensive, but oh boy, does it deliver. It takes a little time to see the effect, but you can add coat after coat which builds to a gorgeous, thick, black, full-looking finish. It gives a real professional-looking result with no clumps and the result is almost as if you're wearing lash extensions.

Catrice Lash Sensation Definition & Volume Mascara €

Let's leave aside the name, because this product does not live up to it. But it's another super-cheap pick for day – we're more than happy to scrimp on a product for the office and this is it. The brush allows you to get in at small lashes, it doesn't clump and it will give some length and definition.

L'Oréal Paris Volume Million Lashes €€

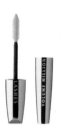

OK, first things first: no, you won't get one million lashes. But you will get a nice medium-thick finish that defines the lash fringe well. The brush is also good and separates well.

Lancôme Hypnôse Drama €€€

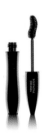

Va va voom! This is seriously volumising and lengthening and it gives the most gorgeous result that's perfect for night-time drama. You quite literally cannot part us from this. It can be slightly messy on the lids, but for such a good result, we don't mind.

Clinique High Lengths €€

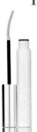

Totally one of our favourite mascaras of recent years. Yes, the wand is weird, but that's why it works. You can get this right into the base of the lashes and the teeny tines coat and define each lash really well. Brilliant!

L'Oréal Paris Telescopic Explosion €€

The mad-looking small round spiky brush is a bit scary, but it's precise, allowing you to get in at all the small lashes at the sides of the eyes and on the lower lash line. It's great for depth of colour and volume. You need a steady hand with this one – it's all too easy to poke yourself in the eye, so beware!

Estée Lauder Sumptuous Extreme Lash Multiplying Mascara €€€

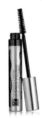

A real old-school mascara, this. It's good and weighty, a pleasure to apply, clean mascara, defines well and perfect for daytime eyes. No flakes down your face either.

Max Factor Masterpiece Max €€

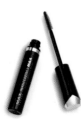

An old reliable, this is a mid-priced classic that's stood the test of time. Gives fab volume, doesn't smudge or budge and is much copied, which kinda says it all really!

Bourjois 1001 Lashes Black Quartz €€

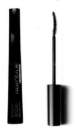

A good pick for day, this is a basic mascara with a new-gen wand. It doesn't do anything major in the volumising or lengthening stakes but does give some definition and fans the lash fringe out nicely.

Maybelline Lash Stiletto €€

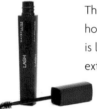

This defines lashes really well without any gunky clumps or horrid stuck-together spider's legs. Its main achievement though is lengthening: it's not very volumising, but it gives a definite extension to the length of lashes.

Clinique Lash Building Primer €€

This is a good way to get extra drama from a disappointing mascara. Whack a coat of this on first, let it dry for a few seconds and then apply your regular product on top. *Voilà!* A souped-up result – we like.

La Roche-Posay Densifying Mascara €€

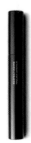

Great for those with sensitive eyes or for contact lens wearers, this is a really kind and gentle mascara. It's also got nourishing goodies in it that promote the growth of healthy, strong lashes.

Cult Product: Chanel Inimitable Intense €€€

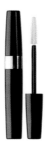

It's oh so chic, darlings, and a rare case where the sequel is better than the original. Rich and dark, it somehow manages to curl lashes upwards in the most flattering way, opening up the eye while dramatising the lashes. The brush is great, simple and sleek and dispenses an even amount of mascara without the dreaded clumping.

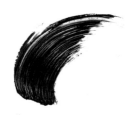

Psst: Heard About the Wand Wizard?

One of the funniest pieces of industry news we've heard was the admission that the L'Oréal group is so committed to produce the best mascara result in the whole universe that they employ someone whose sole job is to develop new mascara wands. They call him the Wand Wizard. Take that, Harry Potter!

Mascara Wardrobe

By now many of us are familiar with the concept of a fragrance wardrobe: having a collection of different perfumes to suit different moods and occasions. But a mascara wardrobe? Having a different mascara to suit different moods? It brings to mind a vision of tiny wardrobes filled with tubes (and in my case a good few fecked on the floor, having fallen off their hangers).

Although it initially sounds like a bit of a ridiculous ploy, we have given it some consideration and think it may actually be something that many of us do anyway.

● Reason for Mascara Wardrobe #1

Most women have a few mascaras anyway. Like lip gloss, they are cheap and easy to pick up and – this is key – easy to lose, so you require a constant influx into the wardrobe.

● Reason for Mascara Wardrobe #2

Sometimes you will want a subtle look and sometimes you will require a mascara with a little more impact. Equally, sometimes you want length and separation and sometimes you want volume more than anything. Sadly, we haven't yet come across one mascara that does all these things really well, so you really do need at least two. We swear.

● Reason for Mascara Wardrobe #3

You're conducting serious scientific research. Mascara science is a wonderful thing and has given us lengthening fibres, rotating and vibrating wands, serum-imbued growth enhancers as well as black gunk the colour of priests' socks. It's research, owning a wardrobe of 'em, honest.

Hot Stuff

Has your mascara gone all hard and gunky? Give it a new lease on life by placing the entire tube (with lid tightly closed) in a cup of hot water for a couple of minutes before you apply.

Brows

Honestly, getting and maintaining a good brow shape is one of the best things you can do for your beauty routine. We love the service at Estée Lauder Brow Bars and we also highly rate threading as a first fix. Then once brows are at their best, you can maintain them at home with these top product picks.

Tip Don't Over-pluck

We used to be obsessed with our brows, plucking each and every day in a frantic effort to keep them looking great. But we were actually over-plucking and after a conversation with an expert who advised us that this can lead to bald patches in later life, we eased up. It's incredibly common for girls to pluck like crazy in their twenties, only to find that once their forties hit, oestrogen production has dropped and with that can come balding brows. So keep them tidy by all means, but don't be too over-zealous unless you're happy to draw in your eyebrows in years to come.

Recommendations

Shop Smart: Essence Eyebrow Stylist Set €

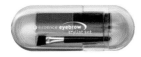

This kit contains two powder shadows, three brow shape templates and a little brush. A great first buy for anyone just getting into brow shaping and definition who doesn't want to shell out big bucks on a product from Benefit or Urban Decay.

Clarins Eyebrow Kit Pro €€€€

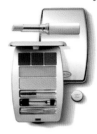

Clarins Eyebrow Kit Pro is fab. Three powder colours to suit all hair shades, wax, a pink powder to brighten under-brow skin and three teeny tools to tweeze, tidy and apply. Ace.

Artdeco Eye Brow Colour Pen €€

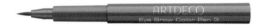

One for those who have lost brows due to illness or over-plucking, this marker-like pen allows you to literally draw hairs, in feather-light strokes, to mimic the appearance of brows.

Clinique Instant Lift for Brows €€

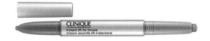

This double-ended doofer is a very handy thing to have in your kit. A coloured wax nib on one end lets you fill in and shape brows and a creamy highlighter on the other end can be used to add definition under the brow. We're not mad on that part of it, but the wax works very well.

Cult Product: Tweezerman Tweezers €€€

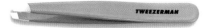

We've tried many tweezers over the years and the one we come back to time and time again is that old faithful, Tweezerman. Available in a baffling array of colours, tip types and handle lengths, these reliable yokes are an easily available beauty staple and something every girl needs to own.

Powder Shadow

Don't feel like you absolutely need to shell out on a dedicated brow product. You don't – powder shadow works just as well to shape and fill in sparse brows. Lightly apply with a small angled brush in the direction of the hair growth and Bob's yer uncle. If you need to, you can set it with a tiny (we mean tiny) amount of clear Vaseline on an old, clean mascara wand.

Nails

Nails are without doubt the biggest area of excitement and creativity we've seen in the last couple of years and it's a trend that just keeps growing legs. Each new colour and shade is eagerly anticipated and we've got our eyes on the catwalk months ahead so we can see what shades are going to be hot next season. Duping is particularly strong in this category, and for that we say yay, because it saves us lots and lots of cash.

Trend: Nail Art and Embellished Nails

Previously the province of trained experts, the availability of affordable nail art pens from Models Own and nail decals and tip guides from Essence means we can all get down with nail art ourselves, and for really affordable prices. Sadly, the one thing we can't buy is a steady hand.

Stickey Sandwich €€

A brilliant way to keep your mani in place for longer, the Stickey sandwich consists of several layers of polish and CND's cult Stickey Base Coat. Lash it on first, then a layer of colour. Apply a second coat of Stickey, another layer of colour and a top coat. Let it dry and you should have a set of decorated digits that are pretty much bomb proof.

Beaut.ienomics:
Make Nails Your Recession Treat

Nails are one of the biggest and best recession-busting beauty treats out there. Transformative and fun, you don't have to spend a lot because budget brands offer brilliant choice and allow you a beauty spree for just a few quid. A perfectly painted set of nails lifts anyone's spirits and you can have fun with them too – create an accent nail, match your lips to your tips or experiment with glitter and different coloured French tips. It really is the beauty bit you can indulge in no matter how tight your budget.

Recommendations

Shop Smart: Essence €

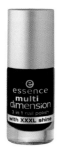

This budget brand has a huge selection of different nail varnish options, from tiny little bottles of flouro polishes to bigger vials of smoky greys, taupes, darks, pastels and brights. You'll always find something to mimic a trend for a tiny price, which pleases us greatly.

CND Stickey Base Coat €€

This base coat grips colour coats and definitely helps to keep them in place longer. Try using it in between coats of polish too for the infamous 'Stickey sandwich' (see p. 190)!

Nubar €

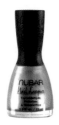

Nubar is a professional range available at salons, but unlike most salon ranges it's affordable, at less than a tenner a bottle. Importantly, it's 3 free – no nasties like formaldehyde and a couple of other things we can't pronounce. There's a great range of shades and good lasting power. (For more on 3 free, see p. 197.)

Gosh €

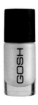

Great shades and affordable prices are the reasons why we like Gosh's varnishes so much. Nice thin formulations and quirky little products like holographic polishes make it a fun range too.

Barry M €

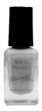

When these are on three for two at Boots, we snap them up. Brilliant at brights and copying seasonal trend shades, Barry M polishes have good longevity too.

OPI €€

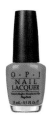

The bee's knees of polish brands, OPI releases a myriad of collections each year based around all sorts of themes and celebrities. Because it's a salon range, there's a huge shade choice, which helps to justify the more expensive price. Plus you've got lots of formulation options, like glitter or matte.

Models Own €

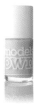

You can't beat this brand for its ability to copy catwalk trends in a jiffy. There's a huge variety on offer too: glitters, shimmers, crèmes and all manner of fancy top coats abound. The thin formulas dry really quickly and allow you to lash on two or three coats quickly.

Bourjois €

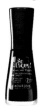

We particularly like the So Laque polishes because they're so easy to use. One coat's usually enough, there's an excellent shade choice, they dry quickly and the brush makes application simple.

Rimmel 60 Seconds €

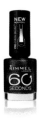

60 Seconds is fantastic and it really does dry quickly. The brush is a really nice fat shape and paints each nail with one stroke. Loads of 'fashion colours' (God we sound like *Woman's Own* here, but it's true) are available and the polish is thick, meaning you can often get away with just one coat.

Chanel €

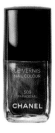

Chanel's fab shades are irresistable. This brand always sets the bar and then the budget brands rush in to copy its colours. So if you want to be first, queue up for Chanel, but if you're not fussed about the brand you use, check the duping section (pp. 127–8) for inspiration.

The Nail Doctor Dry It You'll Like It €

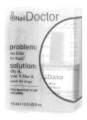

Put a drop of this over each wet nail and they'll be rock hard in seconds. This is fab to have on hand when you're in a hurry or can't be bothered waiting for your manicure to set.

Essence French Manicure Tip Guides €

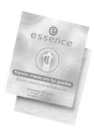

The classic French mani is not in fashion right now, but we do like creating different coloured tips and half-moons down by the cuticle and these cheap little fellers are great, helping you to get sharp, clean edges.

Leighton Denny Crystal Nail File €€

A real can't-live-without, this file is expensive, but it will last you years. Glass files make shaping a cinch and also help to seal the tip of the nail, which helps prevent weak, flaky nails. And if it gets a bit clogged, run it under some warm water and pat dry with a towel.

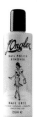

L'Onglex Nail Polish Remover €

This takes even the darkest varnish off easily and quickly, therefore it's good for the environment too, as you use fewer cotton pads! The oily formula means it's kind to nails – acetone free is the kindest.

Cult Product: Seche Vite Dry Fast Top Coat €€

Not just a cult product, this one goes stellar. It's the top coat no nailista can live without, trust us. No chips, dries fast – this is pure magic for manicures. Like the thought of lashing two layers of polish straight on top of a base coat and then running out the door five minutes later? So do we, and with Seche Vite, we can.

Try Something New

There's lots more nail fun than mere polish available. The past couple of years have seen the rise of increasingly good three-week manicures like Shellac, which is a great bet if you like to paint and go. Offering lots of colours and finishes, it looks like regular polish, is super-shiny and sticks about for ages.

Nail wraps like Minx have only added to the fun. You can choose from a bewildering array of patterned and metallic decals that are then heated onto nails and should stay put for about a week. And of course, where one innovates, others follow – check out Essence's super-cheap nail wraps for a fun take on the trend.

Stick-on nails have come on in leaps and bounds too. No longer limited to a set of French-tipped Broadways, now you can buy all sorts of adhesive nails with patterns, glitter and colour pre-painted on. They're great fun and brilliant for immediate impact.

Plus, salon manicures are now really affordable for a basic file and paint, meaning we can indulge occasionally even when we're not feeling so flush.

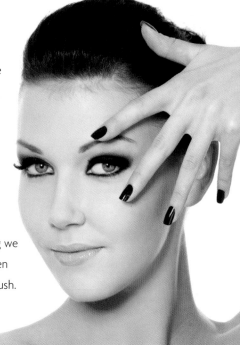

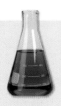

Read the Ingredients

Ingredient watching is a particularly hot topic among nail fans these days and all the hippest lines proclaim themselves '3 free'. Basically, what this means is that polish with this label won't have the chemical nasties formaldehyde, dibutyl phthalate (DBP) and toluene in it. Buying 3 free means your polish will be kinder to your nails, and hey, we all like a bit of that. Brands to try include Orly, Butter London and Nubar.

Wah! Why Doesn't My Polish Stay Put?

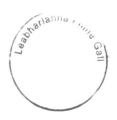

Use Cuticle Oil

A lot of the time the reason lacquer flakes is because nails are weak and flexible. The best thing to do in this case is to keep them short and well filed and don't over-buff. Try a daily cuticle oil too, which can strengthen them from the base. We like CND's SolarOil and Essie Apricot Cuticle Oil.

Notes

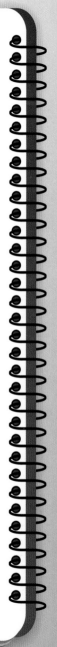

Notes

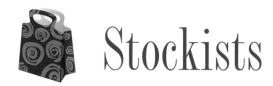

Stockists

- **Armani, Giorgio cosmetics**, at Brown Thomas Dublin and Cork and Dublin Airports
- **Aveda**, at Brown Thomas, House of Fraser and Whetstone salons; at Carton House spa, Maynooth
- **Aveeno**, at supermarkets

- **Babyliss**, at Argos and department stores
- **Barbara Daly**, at Tesco stores nationwide
- **Benefit**, at department stores nationwide
- **Barry M**, at Superdrug stores and selected Boots
- **Bobbi Brown**, at Brown Thomas branches
- **Body Shop**, stores nationwide
- **Bourjois**, at chemists and Boots

- **Catrice**, at Dunnes and pharmacies
- **Cetaphil**, at pharmacies
- **Chanel**, at department stores and good chemists
- **Clarins**, at pharmacies and department stores
- **Clinique**, at department stores nationwide and good chemists
- **Crème de la Mer**, at Brown Thomas, Harvey Nichols Dundrum and Dublin Airport

- **Dermalogica**, at salons nationwide, 1850 556 785
- **Dior cosmetics**, at department stores and selected pharmacies
- **Dove**, at supermarkets and pharmacies

- **Elemis**, at department stores, chemists and spas nationwide
- **Elizabeth Arden**, at department stores nationwide and selected pharmacies

- **Essence Cosmetics**, at Dunnes, Penneys, Heatons and pharmacies
- **Essie**, at selected salons nationwide
- **Estée Lauder**, at department stores nationwide and selected pharmacies
- **Eucerin**, at pharmacies

- **Garnier**, at supermarkets and pharmacies
- **Giorgio Armani cosmetics**, at Brown Thomas Dublin and Cork and Dublin Airports

- **Inglot**, Unit 23A (beside Starbucks), Liffey Valley

- **John Frieda**, at supermarkets and chemists

- **Kerastase**, at L'Oréal Professionel salons, including Peter Mark branches
- **Kiehl's**, Wicklow Street, Dublin 2, 01 670 6667

- **La Roche-Posay**, at chemists nationwide
- **Lancôme**, at department stores and pharmacies
- **Lavera**, at health food stores nationwide
- **Liz Earle**, QVC Beauty, www.lizearle.com and Wilde & Green, Miltown, Dublin 6
- **L'Occitane**, branches nationwide, www.loccitane.com
- **L'Onglex**, available nationwide at Dunnes, Superquinn, Spar and lots of smaller outlets
- **L'Oréal Paris**, at chemists and supermarkets

- **MAC**, at Brown Thomas, selected BT2 stores and Dublin Airport
- **Make Up For Ever**, 40 Clarendon Street, Dublin 2, 01 679 9043 and Arnotts, Henry Street, Dublin 1
- **Maybelline**, at chemists and supermarkets
- **Max Factor**, at chemists and Debenhams branches

- **Models Own**, at Boots (**NI:** Ballymena; Boucher Rd, Belfast; Sprucefield, Lisburn; Derry; Coleraine. **ROI:** Jervis; Stephen's Green, Half Moon Street, Cork; Swords, Co. Dublin) as well as Asos.com, Modelsownit.com and selected River Island stores
- **MoroccanOil**, at Zeba, Dylan Bradshaw, Queen Beauty Emporium

- **NARS**, at Brown Thomas Dublin
- **Neutrogena**, at chemists, supermarkets and Boots nationwide
- **Nivea**, at supermarkets
- **Nubar**, at salons and online
- **Nuxe**, Arnotts, Clerys and pharmacies nationwide

- **Olay**, at supermarkets
- **OPI**, at salons and leading pharmacies
- **Organic Surge**, Boots Liffey Valley, Clerys, Dunnes, Hickeys, McCabes and Unicare pharmacies as well as independent pharmacies nationwide
- **Origins**, at Arnotts, Clerys, House of Fraser, Boots Liffey Valley and Dublin Airport

- **Pantene**, at supermarkets and pharmacies

- **Queen Beauty Emporium**, 66-67 Aungier St, Dublin 2, 01 478 9633

- **REN,** at Clerys, Alchemist Earth or call 01 461 0645
- **Revlon**, at larger Boots stores (including Liffey Valley), Debenhams branches and independent pharmacies nationwide
- **Revlon Professional**, 01 886 9300
- **Rimmel**, at supermarkets and pharmacies
- **RoC**, at pharmacies nationwide
- **Roger & Gallet**, at pharmacies, 1890 812 741

- **Smashbox**, at chemists nationwide
- **Soap & Glory**, at Harvey Nichols, Dundrum and larger Boots stores
- **Strivectin**, at Arnotts and Harvey Nichols, Dundrum
- **St Tropez**, at department stores and pharmacies

- **Tom Ford fragrance and cosmetics**, at Brown Thomas Dublin and selected fragrance items at Harvey Nichols
- **Trilogy**, at Arnotts in Dublin, select pharmacies and health stores nationwide, including Nourish, Unicarepharmacy and www.safiaorganics.ie. For a full list of stockists, visit trilogyproducts.com.

- **Urban Decay**, at selected Boots, Debenhams and House of Fraser stores; Debenhams Dublin, Cork, Belfast, Blanchardstown, Foyleside, Limerick, Newbridge and Cara and Neary's Pharmacy.

- **Vichy**, at pharmacies nationwide

- **Yves Saint Laurent Beaute**, at department stores, including Brown Thomas and Arnotts

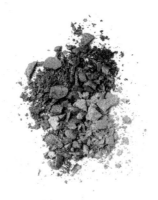

Index